DISTRESS IN THE CITY

DISTRESS
IN
THE CITY

ESSAYS ON THE DESIGN AND
ADMINISTRATION OF URBAN
MENTAL HEALTH SERVICES

Edited by William Ryan
With an Introduction by Erich Lindemann

The Press of Case Western Reserve University
Cleveland and London · 1969

CONTENTS

v

PART THREE
A New Mental Health Agenda—William Ryan

LIST OF TABLES

PREFACE

In a very important sense, this book is a product of the Boston Mental Health Survey, initiated in the fall of 1960 and completed in the summer of 1962. In the rapidly changing world of mental health, that was a long time ago: before the state planning projects, before the federal community mental health center program, and long before the Comprehensive Health Planning Program.

And the Boston survey itself had forbears: a committee appointed by United Community Services of Metropolitan Boston, chaired by Dr. Gerald Caplan, that was given the charge of assessing the problems of coordinating mental health services in Greater Boston.

I feel impelled at least to mention the names of some of the many persons who contributed to this long, time-linked process that began ten, twenty, even thirty years ago in Boston (there was a survey in the late 1930's of the Boston mental health scene).

There were three agencies co-sponsoring the Boston survey—the Massachusetts Department of Mental Health, the United Community Services of Metropolitan Boston, and the Massachusetts Association for Mental Health. Staff members of these agencies constituted a Steering Committee for the Survey—Dr. B. R. Hutcheson, Dr. Carola Blume, and Arthur Hallock (Department of Mental Health); Edward Kovar, Leo Friel, Robert Ott, and Mrs. Ledonia Wright (United Community Services); Dr.

Lynn Beals, Dr. Libbie Bower, and Edith Abraams (Massachusetts Association for Mental Health)—and they shared in the ultimate responsibility for the shape and conduct of the survey. Their planning for the survey was substantially aided by consultation from Dr. Reginald Robinson, now Executive Director of the Massachusetts Committee on Children and Youth. In addition to her role as a member of the Steering Committee, Mrs. Wright's contribution to the collection and analysis of data for the survey was extremely helpful.

The principal staff members of the survey were Dr. Franklin Fogelson, now with the University of Maryland; Dr. Edward O'Donnell, now with the Department of Health, Education and Welfare; and Mrs. Maria Levinson. Dr. Fogelson did a preliminary study of the referral process of mental health problems; Dr. O'Donnell conducted an extremely significant study of the relationship between personal and community values and mental health planning and programming in two Boston communities. His study was not reported in the survey summary but is available in his doctoral dissertation.[1] Mrs. Levinson took primary responsibility for the design and execution of the referral study reported in some detail in Part One of this book. The formulations and insights which she developed provide a major theme both for the report of the original survey and for many of the commentaries in Part Two. Her contribution to the Boston survey was invaluable.

The Advisory Committee to the Survey was composed of a number of very dedicated and very busy citizens of Boston, who gave freely of their time and energy to counsel and assist the staff during the conduct of the survey itself, to derive the important implications that lay unseen within the data, and, after the completion of the survey, to push Boston and Boston's agencies to recognize and confront the many tasks that were made more

---

[1] Edward O'Donnell, "Community Value Orientations and Mental Health." (Ph.D. dissertation, Brandeis University, 1965).

evident by the work of the survey. Mrs. Catherine Driscoll was Chairman of the Advisory Committee and in this instance, as in so many other instances when there was a need for someone to speak to Boston's human service agencies in the name of the consumers of those services, she acted with her customary intelligence, compassion, and tact. Mr. Maurice Lazarus served as chairman of a subcommittee that worked on the derivation of implications and recommendations from the survey data. Other members of the Advisory Committee included the late Abbie Dunks, the late Dr. Kenneth Wollan, Dr. Austin Berkeley, Dr. Gerald Caplan, Howard Doyle, Mrs. Barbara Elam, Dr. Robert Freckleton, Dr. Frederick Gillis, Rabbi Roland Gittelsohn, Rita Kelleher, Msgr. Francis Lally, Charles Liddell, Dr. Erich Lindemann, Donald Moreland, Paul O'Friel, Dr. Eveoleen Rexford, Judge David Rose, Bishop Anson Phelps Stokes, and Dr. Arthur Tyler.

A sequel to the Boston survey was the Mental Health Planning Committee of Metropolitan Boston, sponsored by the three agencies that had planned the survey itself. This committee was established in the spring of 1965, initially under the leadership of Dr. Erich Lindemann and subsequently of Dr. Sprague Hazard. Its members have been striving mightily to deal with the problems made visible by the survey, but they have been handicapped both by lack of resources and by a real lack of sanction to undertake comprehensive planning. One of their activities was the publication and distribution of the summary report of the survey, which now constitutes Part One of this book.

The final links in the sequence require a few more acknowledgments. The survey report was circulated without publicity, but two informal advocates were instrumental in bringing it to the attention of many people. They were Dr. Donald Kenefick, Associate Director of the National Association for Mental Health, and Dr. George Albee, who has also contributed a wise and pointed chapter to Part Two of this book.

And, of course, following this long story with patience, support, and much love have been my wife, Phyllis, and my daughter, Elizabeth, to whom are dedicated my contributions to this book. To my wife, in particular, I wish to express my loving thanks for her support, her encouragement, and her wise and trenchant counsel.

New Haven, Connecticut
December 5, 1968

INTRODUCTION

This volume deals with one of the most important problems of contemporary community life: the provision of appropriate services for individuals in emotional distress. A survey of the deployment of professional resources in outpatient clinics, child guidance centers, and casework agencies that was executed by Dr. Ryan in Boston serves as a point of departure for a penetrating discussion by a group of distinguished members of the professions engaged in research and service in psychiatry, psychology, and the wide field of social welfare. They not only review and appraise the facts elicited in this survey but also address themselves to possible causes of the inadequacies of professional services and suggest several approaches for remedial planning.

It will be seen that this survey, which was initiated by a committee and which brought together for joint planning professionals from the fields of psychiatry, psychology, and social work, board members of agencies, and representatives of the state Department of Mental Health, was intended at first to provide material for more effective cooperation between all those concerned with the care and early discovery of emotional disturbances. However, the conceptualization and execution of the study had the precision and clarity which invites constructive criticism and indicates desirable further investigation in the new field of comparative community studies. Indeed, the survey raises questions about the underlying assumptions that form the basis of much of the ongoing mental health work; and it makes possible the consideration of significant innovations in planning for preventive psychiatry and, far beyond, for new patterns in the organization of the social welfare services now often referred to as "human services," in which the concern with emotional disturbances plays a significant, but not the most important, part.

Dr. Ryan's study became possible because different professional groups, often divided in value priorities and preferences, had decided to seek new ways of cooperation. For a decade it had been clear that any preventive psychiatry of the future would have to be based on the observations and services of many collaborating groups in the community—all the various care-givers who have access to persons at times of severe life crises under the conditions of rapid social change and in the face of social conflict and deprivation. Psychiatrists who are interested in the possible pathological consequences of such critical periods must become acquainted with all those in the community who have access to disturbed persons and who have developed procedures of intervention and helpful assistance. Thus, the clergy at times of bereavement, the teacher confronted with adolescent turmoil, and the social worker in the face of family crisis or economic defeat are all concerned with emotional disturbances that may be precursors of mental illness. The manner in which their helpful intervention may constitute preventive work is beginning to be understood by psychiatrists, but it needs a great deal more research. This psychiatric interest overlaps significantly the concerns of psychologists, who in the field of social psychology look for opportunities to study the dynamics of emotional crises engendered by social conflict and transition. Indeed, psychologists are widening their clinical interests to include the crisis situations in the individual life cycle and in social groups, and they offer a growing body of expertise and social skill to make intervention more effective. Moreover, those professionals who are primarily concerned with social structure and the consequences of certain types of social processes for those individuals who have to live with them are developing new concepts and new organizational practices designed to reduce the number of casualties. What is needed is the development of mutually acceptable and facilitating modes of collaboration in order to widen the segment of the population that can be reached by services and multiply the opportunities to gain new insights in the respective cooperating fields.

This type of collaboration among professional groups is just beginning. One very promising form of communicating with each other and simultaneously with the public is the type of professional exchange presented in this volume.

We are not surprised to find a high level of emotion, emphatic presentation of divergent views, and highly critical comments by professionals from different fields about each other. The flavor of eager and animated controversy is a necessary prelude to finding shared values and concepts acceptable in several fields. Only then can one begin to find mutual accommodations in the redistribution of prerogatives and role assignments for various professional groups in the community.

The factual core of this study is the documentation of inadequate and uneven distribution of services for the emotionally disturbed in a metropolitan area which has an unusually high level of professional resources in psychiatry and clinical psychology as well as social work. It thus makes explicit a state of affairs which implicitly was known or at least guessed at by the members of the advisory committee for the study. In his search for possible causal factors Dr. Ryan extends his review to a description of referral techniques, admission priorities, and styles of intervention. He thus reveals another fact that was informally known—that each professional agency in the course of its development will begin to prefer for admission those patients for whom it seems to represent the highest level of competence in diagnosis and treatment and for whom experience has shown the prospects for therapeutic success to be relatively good. When these agencies were started, they were expected to be examples of highly sophisticated clinical work with a correctly chosen clientele. We sometimes forget how recent is the development of a new value orientation, fostered by those engaged in public mental health, with a concern for populations rather than for individuals. Along with this new perspective goes optimism looking toward tools of intervention on a population-wide basis that may be provided by the social sciences. This orientation is reinforced by the growing quest on the part of the underprivileged and disfranchised for equal participation in the use of community resources and by the growing sense of obligation on the part of the more privileged members of society, including politicians and professionals. We now think not so much about excellent treatment of the individual case as about equal opportunities for all members of the community.

In the light of these values, indeed, what appeared adequate and quite excellent agency performance where only a few clients or patients were concerned now appears highly inadequate and obsolescent because of the failure to reach early a large segment of the community. The survey finds that all these institutions fall far short of serving all their applicants, let alone searching for possible other persons who might need these services, particularly the poor, the aged, and the adolescent.

It might be understandable in the light of our new values that we disapprove of this type of agency operation and castigate the professions involved; and we are apt to forget that these very agencies have established the knowledge about psychodynamics and psychological chains of events that has given rise to our current optimism about crisis intervention. It is equally clear, however, that new designs for collaborative efforts, involving a variety of competences and research methodologies, are needed now. What are some of the questions that arise? Can the psychiatric profession modify its conceptual approach and the perception of its role in the community, and, indeed, is it willing to do so? Perhaps the theoretical framework evolved by psychoanalysis and used in psychotherapy is not suitable for the new tasks. Can psychiatric training be altered to include adequate knowledge of social structure and process and new skills in collaboration with other professions? And can psychiatrists be motivated to relinquish private practice and concern with the privileged for the difficult challenge of communication with the poor and with different ethnic groups? Many signs indicate that indeed they will make concerted efforts in these new directions.

On the other hand, will those professional groups whose primary concern is the community, the social context of living, and the organizational approach to psychosocial problems find the psychiatric contribution still worthwhile, or will they insist on a language incompatible with psychiatric and clinical orientation? Perhaps new forms of social administration are all that is needed, and a new mandate must be given to those professionals seeking a larger part in planning and care for the emotionally disturbed, the handicapped, and the underprivileged. Finally, is it realistic to expect that voluntary agencies with their own histories and their own unique goals can come to an agreement with governmental agencies about collaborative planning of mutually supportive efforts to cover as large a part of the total community as possible? If not, can patterns of legal enforcement be found to guarantee these services? And, indeed, are we prepared at this time with our concepts and methods to accept and sanction any specific pattern of authority and prerogatives? The community mental health centers established by federal law can be most useful here if they provide for careful development and evaluation of different patterns of community care and different ways of aligning mental health issues with those in general health and social welfare.

How near are we to a hopeful level of consensus? There are indeed some areas of agreement among the discussants of the Ryan report. They might be named as follows: First, the conditions described in Boston can safely be considered as typical for the whole nation—for other metropolitan areas, and perhaps even for some rural regions. Second, the problem cannot be solved by a simple increase in professional manpower. Demand will increase with the available supply of services and the resources will always fail to meet the needs. Third, the problem is related to the distribution of human services which excludes from access the poor, the aged, and many persons during transition periods in the life cycle. There is agreement, finally, on the prospect of successful retraining of psychiatrists to assume modified roles as they participate and contribute their psychodynamic insight to joint problem-solving with other professions at the consultation and planning level.

However, there is considerable disagreement about the degree to which psychiatric personnel and institutions should assume responsibility for the revision of mental health services. Much emphasis is placed on the overexpansion of the range of problems for which the psychiatrists consider themselves competent. There is also the feeling that the concepts and orientations stemming from the psychoanalytic period of psychotherapy are unsuitable for meeting the new challenges and should be replaced by concepts developed in the field of learning theory and behavioral approaches to human distress.

A plea is made that psychiatrists should return to the narrower field of clinical concerns and restrict their efforts to established disease, leaving the fields of prevention to those who deal with human behavior on a broader basis, who consider social deviance not in medical but in legal, societal, and value terms, and who concern themselves with disturbed states as categories of *social* disturbance often labeled with the term "alienation." Such a plan would require the invention and implementation of patterns of social organization and community participation, which require primarily, if not exclusively, the services of the social scientists and the social action experts. Those contributors who are con-

cerned with values and moral attitudes are skeptical of any success in persuading the middle-class establishment to refrain from
attempts to pervert mental health services designed to meet the
needs of the poor. Such skepticism, however, leaves room for the
proposition that greater use of nonprofessional, lay resources, and
subprofessional helpers can do much to aid the job of prevention.
The growing use of the mass media to deal constructively with
the presentation of psychiatric problems is only one form of such
community activity.

There is no question in the mind of any of the contributors but
that all new developments should be geared to research and
evaluation—that we are far from understanding some of the most
basic problems, such as the ambiguity between emotional and
situational disability or between emotional disability and the distress signs accompanying even successful adaptation to environmental stress.

While all this reflects concern with long-range, future development, the question may also be asked about the immediate, practical consequences of the findings presented in the report. Our
volume contains an impressive description of a statewide organization of mental health and welfare services in Minnesota, with a
clear mandate and role allocation for the participant agencies
involved, which was strongly influenced by the description of the
relative chaos in Boston. And in Boston itself? An immediate
consequence was the expansion of the original Committee for
Mental Health to review prospective plans for the metropolitan
area in the light of this report. A most significant concurrent set
of events that was initiated by the Department of Mental Health
as part of the implementation of the program of federal community mental health centers brought forth a design for statewide
redistribution of mental health services with auspicious alignment
of the various professions involved and with active citizen participation in each phase of the development of these centers. Much
of this design was then embodied in the new Mental Health Act,

which profoundly altered the patterns of agency distribution and accessibility of care throughout the state. A significant aspect of the services in the metropolitan area is the provision for leadership and continued research on the part of the local universities, with emphasis on continued innovation and evaluation of program and with the expectation of continued intensive collaboration of the psychiatric and medical departments on the one hand and the social science, law, and education departments on the other.

The details of the propositions, documentation, and illustration contributed by the authors of this volume will be studied with keen interest by all those who have responsibility for the development of new programs and also by the many citizens engaged in the confrontation of basic issues in the field of mental health.

Erich Lindemann, M.D., Ph.D.
Stanford University

I
DISTRESS IN THE CITY: A SUMMARY REPORT OF THE BOSTON MENTAL HEALTH SURVEY

WILLIAM RYAN

THE SURVEY
FINDINGS: PROBLEMS,
NUMBERS,
PEOPLE, AND
PLACES

Every big city has tens of thousands of people in distress, people who are handicapped in their struggle for life and happiness by many kinds of emotional disturbance. The Boston Mental Health Survey was conducted to find out what happens to these people —who notices them, who tries to help them, and what becomes of them. In this summary report, some of the important findings of the survey are described and some of the implications of these findings are discussed.

One way in which these findings are reported is by describing some of the emotional problems from which Bostonians suffer. Another is by reporting numbers—the numbers of persons whom the survey sampled and found to be receiving or not receiving adequate help—though it must be pointed out quite clearly that the numbers that will be given are estimates, not precise figures. Finally, the survey findings may be revealed by telling what happens to emotionally disturbed persons—where they seek help and whether they get it, what kinds of agencies and people are available to give help, and what channels exist in the community by which people can be referred from the place where they are recognized as disturbed to the place where they can get help.

3

In this first part of the report, then, the findings will be organized in four major sections: *problems, numbers, people* (those seeking and offering help), and *places* (agencies and institutions which offer services to the emotionally disturbed). In the second part of the report an attempt will be made to interpret the findings, to bring out some of the implications, to generalize about some of the major problems and barriers existing within Boston's network of mental health services, and to offer a major proposal for action.

I. Problems

In order to make sense of the survey findings, it is first necessary to have some grasp of the general subject matter—emotional disturbance—and, most important, of the kinds of human beings with whom the survey was concerned—emotionally disturbed persons. Much has been written about, and many attempts have been made to define, mental health and mental illness. It would, of course, be possible to do the same in this report. A different approach has been chosen, however. Rather than definitions, the cases of actual persons, possessing a variety of different problems, will be presented. It is hoped that through this method the reader will be able to deduce for himself a meaningful sense of the range of behavior under consideration.

In general, it can be said that in this report the category of "emotionally disturbed person" covers more of us than those persons who might be labeled "psychotic" or "insane" and far fewer of us than those persons who deviate somewhat from a hypothetical standard of "good mental health" or the state of being "well-adjusted." The category does include those whose emotional disturbance is of sufficient magnitude to interfere to an obvious degree with normal functioning. On the basis of recent studies of urban populations, such as the *Midtown Manhattan*

Study,[1] it appears that this criterion covers between 20 and 25 per cent of the population.

WHAT IS AN EMOTIONALLY DISTURBED PERSON?

The term "emotionally disturbed person" has different meanings to different individuals. It has never been so well defined that it has a common meaning everywhere. *For the Boston Mental Health Survey an emotionally disturbed person was defined as one who is in some sense handicapped by emotional disturbance* —for example, a person who is not able to work as effectively as he might or who has difficulties getting along with other persons or in carrying out family responsibilities. The range of symptoms which can be included in the broad category of emotional disturbance is wide. Emotional disturbance may show itself in irritability and quick temper, in withdrawal from and disinterest in other persons, or in some kind of physical symptom, such as a headache or a stomachache. It may show itself in unusual behavior, such as when a young boy gets in a lot of fights or a grown man moves from one job to another for no apparent reason. Sexual activity may reveal emotional disturbance: a young girl may be unable to bear a man's hand on her arm, or at the opposite extreme a young man may be unable to feel that he is a man unless he has frequent intercourse with casually met strangers. At the outer limits of severe emotional disturbance, behavior is recognized by almost everyone as being "crazy." A person then is seen as so disturbed that he is "out of his mind."

The common dimension of significant emotional disturbance is that of handicap. An emotional handicap is of concern to the community when it significantly interferes with a person's ability

---

[1] There are two volumes in this study: Leo Srole *et al., Mental Health in the Metropolis: The Midtown Manhattan Study* (New York: McGraw-Hill, Inc., 1962); and Thomas S. Langner and Stanley T. Michael, *Life Stress and Mental Health* (Glencoe, Illinois: The Free Press, 1963).

to live his life effectively, and this is the dimension that was used to define emotional disturbance for purposes of collecting data for the Boston Mental Health Survey.

CASES

Examples of emotionally disturbed persons can be cited from the case material collected during the course of the survey. Of course, details of the individual cases described below have been changed to conceal the identity of the living Bostonians who are described.

A Boy Fails in School

The mother of a twelve-year-old boy, the oldest of three children, came to her family doctor very tense and very worried about her son. The boy was a bright young man who in previous years had done exceptionally well in school. This year his report cards were covered with "D's" and "F's." Discussion with the teacher confirmed the mother's opinion of her son's ability. The teacher believed the boy's problem was not one of intellectual capacity and suggested that perhaps some personal difficulty was interfering with his ability to study and learn in school. The physician heard the story and, since he knew the young man himself, was quick to agree with the teacher's point of view.

This is a typical example of the process of identifying an emotionally disturbed person.

A Girl Can't Get Along

As another example, a twelve-year-old girl had been coming for several years to a community center. Workers at the center had come to know her quite well and over these years had grown more and more worried about her emotional well-being. A consistent pattern had emerged during a three-year period: the girl would become involved in groups—on the playground, in a friendship club, in a sewing class—and after a few weeks would begin to quarrel with the other girls. Soon there would be overt fighting and screaming and, abruptly, she would storm out of the group. In three years the girl had enacted a dozen of these highly emotional "quitting scenes." Almost always, shortly after the scene a staff member would find the girl in a corner, crying bitterly and inconsolably, insisting that all the girls hated her, that they "ganged up" on her, and that nobody wanted to be her friend. By inquiring in the community, staff members of the center discovered that there were many problems in this girl's home. She was the oldest of five children, two of whom were still infants. Her father had been out of work many times in the past five years. He drank heavily and, when he was drunk, fought viciously with his wife. During the past three years the parents had separated four times.

A Woman Grows Old

At the opposite extreme on the age scale was a fifty-eight-year-old housewife with two married children. She had visited her doctor frequently in recent weeks with a number of complaints: she found it difficult to fall asleep at night and to wake up in the morning; she believed that she was losing weight; she had frequent attacks of nausea. During the day she was constantly fatigued, even when she had taken a nap. The doctor talked with her husband, who reported that his wife had become extremely irritable lately and did not seem to be the same person she was a year ago. He was very worried about her inability to get pleasure out of life. He was also concerned to some extent (although he said this was secondary) about her inability to take care of the house, even with only the two of them living there now. The doctor examined her completely and carried out laboratory tests which reassured him that there was no physical basis for the complaints. He therefore concluded that her illness was a manifestation of emotional disturbance.

A Young Woman Is Lonely

A thirty-year-old single girl, employed as a laboratory technician in a general hospital, came to a psychiatrist who was on the teaching staff of the hospital where she worked. She reported that she had just broken her engagement and that this was the third time in the past seven years she had broken with a man whom she had been planning to marry. Three days before, she had celebrated her thirtieth birthday, feeling alone and unloved, very conscious that she was eight hundred miles from her home and her family. As she sat through the evening alone in her apartment, she had suffered an intense sense of dread and foreboding. Her hands shook, she sweated profusely, and later she sank into a state of severe depression that lasted for several hours. At about two o'clock in the morning she seriously thought about killing herself. After several days of thinking about this experience and of looking back on what had been, in the main, an unhappy ten years, she concluded that there was something wrong with her emotionally and she was now seeking help.

Every Person Is Different

These examples can be multiplied many times. More extreme and dramatic cases can be cited: the young man who, instead of sitting in his room and thinking about suicide, climbs to the top of the tallest building in town and threatens to destroy himself in the public view of thousands; the young boy whose disturbance is manifested not by failing grades but by setting fires in his neighborhood; the young girl who not only cannot get along with youngsters her own age but begins to display her disturbance in flagrantly promiscuous sexual behavior. At the core of all these problems are feelings of distress—feelings of anxiety, of depression, of inability to cope with life's problems. And accompanying all these problems is a degree of crippling—emotional crippling that interferes with the major functions of human life.

II. Numbers

When we try to deal with the problem of emotional disturbance quantitatively, when we count and add and divide and report our findings in a series of numbers, it must be remembered that the units we are talking about are distressed persons such as those just described. How much emotional disturbance is there in Boston? How many distressed and handicapped persons?

HOW MANY ARE EMOTIONALLY DISTURBED?

Imagine a group of 1,000 Bostonians, a real cross section of the 700,000 people who live in the city. This group would be made up of all kinds of people—old men and teenagers, married couples, young men on their first jobs, babies, college girls—and they would come from all over the city—Brighton, West Roxbury, Back Bay, the South End, Charlestown. Among this sample of 1,000 Bostonians it is probable that between 200 and 250, or about one out of every four or five, would have emotional problems interfering with their lives, handicapping them in their work, in their social relationships, and in dealing with members of their own families. These problems would range from being nervous and making mistakes when the boss looked over one's shoulder all the way to believing that the Communists were influencing one's thoughts with atomic machines.

Relatively few people would be in the latter category (the overtly psychotic), while large numbers would be found in the ranks of the moderately disturbed, people whose anxiety or hostility interfered with their work, caused quarreling and unhappiness in their marriages, made life difficult for them and made it unpleasant for others to live, work, and play with them.

HOW MANY FIND HELP?

What happens to such disturbed people? Who knows about them? Who tries to help them? From our survey findings (as

TABLE 1. ESTIMATED * DISTRIBUTION OF IDENTIFIED
EMOTIONALLY DISTURBED PERSONS IN BOSTON: TOTAL
NUMBERS AND NUMBERS OF BOSTON RESIDENTS ONLY.

	TOTAL NUMBER IN BOSTON FACILITIES, INCLUDING NON-BOSTONIANS.		NUMBER OF BOSTON RESIDENTS ONLY.	
1. Identified as Emotionally Disturbed....................	280,000		95,000	
2. Number Served.................	167,000		58,000	
3. Distribution of Persons in Different Service Settings:				
a. Treated by nonpsychiatric physicians.................145,000			45,000	
b. Treated in social and community agencies......... 11,000			7,000	
c. Treated in mental health settings:.................. 11,000			6,000	
(1) Mental hospitals........		5,000		4,000
(2) Outpatient clinics.......		3,500		1,200
(3) Private practice........		2,500		800
d. Total number treated.......167,000			58,000	

* The reader is again cautioned that the numbers in this table are compiled
from *estimates* made by reporting agencies and individuals, rather than from actual
counts, and that in some instances quantities were projected from sample data.
While criteria of internal consistency suggest that the estimates are probably quite
accurate, it is recommended that these statistics be interpreted as indices of general
orders of magnitude rather than as precise data.

summarized in Table 1) it is estimated that about one person out
of every five or six—that is, between 150 and 200 out of our
representative sample of 1,000—is recognized and identified by
someone as being emotionally disturbed. This recognition and
identification may be done by a teacher, by a social worker, or by
a clergyman. Great numbers of people are identified by their
family physicians. Relatively few of those who are identified as
emotionally disturbed ever find their way into the city's mental
health facilities—the outpatient clinics, the mental hospitals, and
the offices of private psychiatrists. Of the approximately 150

emotionally disturbed persons who are identified in each thousand of the population only *one* will ultimately find himself being treated in a psychiatrist's office. There will be another eight, perhaps nine, who will apply for help to one of the many outpatient psychiatric clinics in Boston, and of these eight or nine perhaps four will be accepted for treatment. Only two of the four will stay in treatment for more than a few weeks. In addition, another five or six persons will be so disturbed, will behave so bizarrely, and will be so bereft of support from the world around them that admission to a mental hospital will seem to be the only solution for their problems.

To summarize, then: more than 150 persons out of every 1,000 Bostonians are identified as handicapped by emotional disturbance; only 10 of this 150 get help in mental health settings—five go to a mental hospital, four receive treatment in a mental health clinic one is treated by a psychiatrist in private practice.

What of the other 140—what happens to them? By far the largest number—at least two out of five—are taken care of directly by physicians who are not psychiatrists—by family doctors, internists, and pediatricians, either in their private practices or on occasions when they donate their time to the medical outpatient clinics of our large general hospitals. These physicians try to reassure their patients and encourage them to talk a little about their problems. They may offer practical advice and prescribe medication, usually one of the tranquilizing or antidepressant drugs which have been developed in recent years. Prescriptions for such drugs are given to large numbers of persons every year. In Boston our estimates indicate that well over 25,000 people receive such prescriptions each year.

Next to the family doctor, it is found that social agencies and community institutions play the most important role in dealing with emotionally disturbed persons. Casework agencies, settlement houses, churches—these and similar agencies and institutions play a very significant role by using their skills and knowledge in trying to help the emotionally disturbed. Of the 150 disturbed persons in every thousand, approximately 10 are receiving help from one of these sources.

Between medical, social, and mental health resources, we find that about two-thirds of the *identified* emotionally disturbed are being taken care of in some way. They are receiving some kind of help, ranging from intensive psychoanalysis every day for a small handful of people, through weekly interviews with a social worker for a larger number of persons, to occasional counseling with a minister, membership in a golden age club, and tranquilizers from the family doctor. Although only a few are receiving what many consider to be adequate treatment—long-term, once-a-week, intensive psychotherapy—most of the others are getting some kind of attention, some human interest, some support in their struggle with anxiety, unhappiness, and inability to get along with friends and family.

WHAT OF THE OTHERS?

But what of the other one-third, those who have been recognized by a professional person as clearly handicapped by emotional disturbance? What is done for them? In a word—nothing.

For some of these persons, of course, it would be difficult to try to provide help, since they are unsure, or reluctant to admit, that they have a problem or a need for help. But even more important than the question of the motivation of disturbed persons is the issue of resources. Realistically, nothing is "left over" to help this one-third of the disturbed population. There is no place, there are no people, there is no time available to them. It must be remembered also that there are many others *who have not been recognized as disturbed*—probably half again as many as those who have been identified. Most of the persons in this group may not be aware of their need for help and it would be hard to reach them; others may simply not know where to turn to begin the process of seeking help.

These, then, are some of the basic facts, the broad numerical outline of the problem. These numbers represent people, people in need of help for problems of emotional disturbance.

III. People—Seeking and Giving Help

PEOPLE LOOKING FOR HELP

It has been shown both that persons with emotional disturbance —a term covering a wide range of behavior—are identified in many different settings and that there are a number of different courses open to them. A question immediately comes to mind as to what determines the course an emotionally disturbed person will follow in seeking help. Does everyone, for example, have an equal chance of eventually sitting across the desk from a psychiatrist, engaged in a psychotherapeutic interview? Is this selection a random process? It will be recalled that only a tiny percentage of the emotionally disturbed ever receive such treatment. What kinds of people are those who do get to see a private psychiatrist? On the other hand, what kinds of people are those who are identified and treated by the family doctor? Are they different in any way from those who go to a psychiatrist? Similar questions could be asked about other groups, such as those who enter mental hospitals, those who are counseled by clergymen, and those whose treatment takes place in a social casework agency. What are the characteristics of these different groups, and do they differ sharply one from the other?

The survey findings point to distinct differences in characteristics among groups, as shown in Table 2. The differences are evident in factors such as age, sex, social class, type of problem, and place of residence. Some examples of these findings can be summarized to indicate the nature of the differences.

Who Sees the Psychiatrist?

The group with the most clear-cut and distinguishable characteristics is that of persons who go to a psychiatrist. These patients

TABLE 2. CHARACTERISTICS OF DIFFERENT SUBGROUPS OF PATIENTS.*

TYPE OF PATIENT	AVERAGE AGE	RATIO OF MEN TO WOMEN	SOCIAL CLASS LEVEL (INCOME & EDUCATION)	RESIDENCE: RATIO OF HIGHER-SOCIAL-RANK AREAS TO LOWER-SOCIAL-RANK AREAS	TYPES OF SYMPTOMATOLOGY	SOCIAL SITUATION
1. Seen by Private Psychiatrist......29		1:2	High	8:1	Anxiety and depression; only one-fifth severely disturbed.	One-third single, living alone.
2. Seen by Physicians (Private Practice)...39		1:2	Medium	12:1	Tension and depression; one-fifth severely disturbed.	Living in families.
3. Seen by Clergymen....39		1:1	High to Low	1:1	Depression and antisocial behavior; one-third severely disturbed.	Moderate number of broken families and persons living alone.
4. Seen by Group-Work Agencies......13		1:1	Low	1:2	Aggressive or withdrawn behavior, only 5% severely disturbed.	High proportion of broken and disorganized families.
5. Admitted to Mental Hospital......45		1:1	Low	1:5	Bizarre, unrealistic, and severely depressed behavior; one-half not psychotic.	Most never married, living alone in marginal circumstances.

* For numerical estimates (based on responses to survey questionnaires) to which the ratios in this table are related, see the discussion of methodological problems, in Appendix, p. 72.

14

cover a relatively narrow age range, half of them falling between the ages of 22 and 36. About two-thirds are female; four out of five have gone to college or are now college students; and occupations are generally consistent with education, reflecting a class level in the middle and upper ranges. Only about one patient in five is diagnosed by his psychiatrist as psychotic or even borderline psychotic, the great majority being seen as suffering from chronic neurosis or character disorder. Close to half of these patients have had previous psychiatric care. The average patient is described as a person with a chronic character disorder having symptoms reflecting anxiety or depression or both.

Of considerable interest is the unusual residential distribution of these patients. Slightly over half of all Boston residents in private psychiatric treatment live in four contiguous census tracts (out of Boston's 156 census tracts). This area contains less than four per cent of the total Boston population. It is bounded approximately by the Charles River, Boston University, Boylston Street, and the Public Garden. If to this small strip of land is added the rest of Back Bay and the front of Beacon Hill (this enlarged area including about seven per cent of Boston's population), over 70 per cent of all Boston patients in private psychiatric treatment will be included.

It is probable that this residential distribution is partially due to a generalized class factor. It is, after all, necessary to be fairly well off financially in order to afford the fees of a psychiatrist. On the other hand, however, other sections of the city with high social rank (for example, Hyde Park and West Roxbury) contribute only a tiny handful of private patients.

Additional analysis of this interesting phenomenon by the survey staff indicated that, taken as a group, the patients who live in this small strip of the Back Bay are younger, and the ratio of females to males is higher, than in other groupings of private patients by residential area of the city. Four-fifths are female and almost two-thirds are between the ages of 20 and 34. About one-quarter of all Bostonians who are private patients are young women in their twenties and early thirties who live within an area of less than 100 blocks. The total number of young women in this age range (within this 100-block area) is fewer than 6,000, of whom about half have the general educational and economic characteristics of the private patients. In other words, this tiny group of approximately 3,000 young college-educated women in their twenties and early thirties furnishes about one-quarter of the Boston patients in private psychiatric treatment.

Who Goes to the Physician?

This is the largest single group of emotionally disturbed persons. It is estimated that over 60,000 Bostonians a year are identified by family doctors or other nonpsychiatric physicians as being emotionally disturbed. When one looks at the general characteristics of cases reported by physicians in private practice (as compared with cases which might be seen in a clinic, for example), it is found that there is a wide range in terms of age, with the median age being about 40. Approximately one-quarter of the clients are under 20 and about one-fifth are over 60. Women outnumber men by a ratio of two to one. Most clients seem to be of lower-middle-class or middle-class status and tend to live in the better residential districts of the city.

Physicians who have offices in Boston include many suburbanites in their practice. Only about one-third of the patients described in case reports are Bostonians. Most patients live in intact families. The relatively few who do not are usually middle-aged or elderly widows or widowers. The most common type of disorder reported by physicians is anxiety, in the form of either an acute attack or a fairly stable condition. In both cases disturbance is experienced in physical terms—for example, as generalized tension. The next most common category is that of the moderate depressive reaction, again with the disorder being experienced in physical terms, with symptoms such as fatigue and insomnia. Although physicians usually treat these patients themselves with brief counseling and advice and considerable reliance on medication, they tend to refer (usually to a private psychiatrist or, in a few cases, to a psychiatric agency) patients who are psychotic or close to psychotic, particularly if there is evidence of bizarre or peculiar thinking. There also seems to be some tendency to refer patients who behave in an aggressive, antisocial way.

Who Goes to the Clergyman?

The average clergyman sees in his professional capacity twelve to fifteen persons a year whom he judges to be obviously emotionally disturbed. In addition, of course, he recognizes emotional disturbance in many others, but this is the number of people whose disturbance he discovers while acting directly in the role of pastoral counselor. The clergyman himself deals directly with the majority of these clients. He attempts not only to counsel his client but also to help the parishioner to cope more effectively with realistic day-to-day problems of living. Since there are approximately 250 clergymen in the city of Boston,[2] it can be readily calculated that about 3,500 emotionally disturbed persons —almost all residents of Boston—are identified each year by members of this profession. Fewer than a thousand of these persons are referred elsewhere, and these almost always to psychiatric resources. Most of the others the clergyman tries to help himself.

Case studies submitted by clergymen reveal that most clients are in the middle age ranges. Four out of five are between the ages of 20 and 60, and the average age is about 40. There is a slight preponderance of women in this group, and there is some evidence that there is a wide distribution of persons among the

[2] That is, clergymen of the various faiths carrying active responsibility for congregations.

different social classes. This is perhaps to be expected, when one considers that clergymen and their churches are spread rather evenly throughout the city, in both the well-to-do and the poor neighborhoods. About three out of five of these clients are living in intact family situations. Of the remainder about half have been either divorced or widowed and the rest are single persons living alone. The most common types of disturbance reported are described in such a way as to indicate depressive disorders and disorders involving some kind of antisocial behavior on the part of the parishioner. Many of the clients described as depressed and a considerable number of other clients are reported to be thinking, and intensively worrying, about such matters as "personal unworthiness" and "sinfulness." This is not surprising, since presumably the disturbed persons have defined their problems in spiritual terms and consequently have sought a spiritual remedy.

Who Goes to the Group Work Agency?

Executives of group work agencies in Boston estimate that approximately four to five thousand of their clients clearly are emotionally disturbed. They serve directly about three-quarters of these persons, most of whom are teenagers and pre-teenagers. The relatively small number of adults included are reported by workers from settlements rather than from YMCAs or Boys' Clubs. There appears to be a difference in the severity of disturbance in the clientele of these two general categories of group work agencies. The settlements deal with larger numbers of disturbed youngsters than are usually included in the clientele of the Y's and the Boys' and Girls' Clubs. As might be predicted from the location of these agencies, most clients live in disadvantaged neighborhoods and come from working-class families. Almost two-fifths of the families of disturbed clients are actually broken, and in a large proportion of those that are technically intact much disorganization and disruption are manifested. The most common type of disturbance described is aggressive behavior in group situations. A somewhat lesser number of cases is reported in which the basic problem involves difficulty in forming relationships with other children and general social withdrawal. In most cases the degree of disturbance appears to be only moderate; in very few does it seem to be so severe as to approach the borderline or psychotic range.

Who Goes to the Public Mental Hospital?

Over 3,000 Boston residents are admitted to public mental hospitals each year. In this group men outnumber women and patients tend to be in the older age ranges. Only one out of every three to four patients admitted is in the diagnostic category that is usually thought of as the typical one for a psychotic hospitalized patient—that is, the category of schizophrenia. About 20 per cent of the patients are diagnosed as suffering from alcoholism, not usually with sufficient dysfunction to be considered psychotic. In total, not many more than half of the patients admitted are ultimately given a diagnosis of psychosis.

In addition to usually being poor and no longer young, these patients tend to be lacking in environmental supports, often living alone, isolated from any social connections. The majority have never married.

The residential pattern of admissions is also quite striking, showing that the greatest proportion of patients admitted is from those sections of the city that are blighted by poverty, family disorganization, slums, and racial segregation. Middle-class white residential sections of the city tend to have relatively low rates of hospital admissions.

The average length of stay in a public mental hospital is relatively short. The majority of patients are discharged in six months to a year. Because such a high proportion of patients are elderly and suffer from physical brain disorders and other diseases common among the aged, there is a high death rate among admitted patients, up to one out of every five being dead within a year after admission.

THE REFERRAL PROBLEM

As emotionally disturbed persons are identified or begin to seek help on their own, an important social welfare mechanism comes

TABLE 3. ESTIMATED RESULTS OF REFERRAL.

	ESTIMATED TOTAL NUMBER	ESTIMATED NUMBER OF BOSTONIANS
1. Referred By:		
a. Physicians	35,000	12,000
b. Other individuals (clergy & lawyers)	4,500	2,500
c. Agencies and institutions	4,500	3,000
Total	44,000	17,500
2. Referred To:		
a. Psychiatric resources:		
(1) Inpatient	3,000	1,500
(2) Outpatient	27,000	11,000
b. Other resources	14,000	5,000
Total	44,000	17,500
3. Applicants to Outpatient Psychiatric Resources:		
a. Self-referred	3,000	1,000
b. Referred by others	8,000	2,500
Total	11,000	3,500

into play. This is the process of referral, the act of telling a person where he can go to find help and in some way facilitating his access to this source of help.

Estimated statistics on referral, derived from survey data, are summarized in Table 3. It is clear from these findings that the number of emotionally disturbed persons who are involved in some aspect of the referral process is astonishingly high—an estimated total of 44,000, of whom over 17,000 are Boston residents. The great majority of these persons are referred to psychiatric sources of help, usually outpatient facilities or psychiatrists in private practice. Approximately 11,000 Bostonians are directed to outpatient psychiatric resources each year.

Comparison of these estimates with estimates obtained from the outpatient psychiatric resources themselves yields some striking conclusions. Of the 11,000 referred approximately 3,500 Bostonians *apply* to such resources for help. About one-fourth to one-third of these are counted as self-referrals. The remainder, perhaps 2,500, have been referred by others, including friends and other informal sources, as well as by the formal sources of referral upon which we have drawn for our estimates. The comparative estimates, then, indicate that about 11,000 Bostonians are in some sense referred (excluding self-referral) for outpatient psychiatric treatment and that only about 2,500 of them actually apply for such treatment. (Of the estimated *total* number of persons, both residents and non-residents, who are referred— 27,000—a similar proportion—8,000—apply for such care.)

This overall summary would suggest that the referral process tends to be unproductive or inefficient, in that relatively few persons respond to it effectively. It must be remembered, of course, that this summary includes under the term "referral" a variety of different activities, probably ranging from simple information-giving—e.g.: "There is a clinic which helps people with this kind of problem. Why don't you go there?"—to the highly skilled and responsible referral carried out by an experienced professional caseworker. With this point in mind, one of the aims of the Boston Mental Health Survey was to look at the results of referral when it was carried out as a specialized professional social welfare service.

A Referral Follow-up Study

As one part of the Boston survey, a specific referral follow-up study was undertaken. One hundred and forty emotionally dis turbed persons who applied during a defined time-period to two referral resources in Boston for a variety of different kinds of problems and types of assistance were followed up closely to see what actually happened after their contact with the referral bureau. These clients were, for the most part, persons on the lower rungs of the socioeconomic ladder asking for help with problems related to family functioning. They were therefore not wholly representative of the total range of emotionally disturbed persons in the city. On the other hand, they were being serviced by skilled social workers, for whom referral, information-giving, and guidance to persons in trouble and seeking help constitute a major function.

Results of this study were both striking and disconcerting. It was found, for example, that about one-third of the group never approached the agency to which they were referred. Another one-third made some initial contact with the agency, but this contact was broken off after one or two interviews, either as a result of the agency's referring them somewhere else or finding that their problems were not appropriate to its function, or, more frequently, because the client did not return for a scheduled appointment. The small number of clients who were counted as having received significant help as a result of the referral process —the remaining one-third of the total—were by no means provided with all the services required for the problems with which they were coping. In some instances the significant help they received was of a quite limited variety, such as assistance with financial problems. Only a tiny minority of the total group were actually engaged in a helping process related directly to their emotional disturbance.

Why Does the Process Fail?

As a result of analyzing the factors involved in these 140 cases, as well as on the basis of interviews with 20 of these clients one year after they had initially applied for help, it has been possible to derive some suggestive lines of explanation regarding the general failure of the referral process.

1. THE CLASS FACTOR.—First of all, there is a relationship between such factors as education and income level of the client and whether or not he is able to make successful use of the referral process. The more educated, more stably employed client tends to be much more successful in obtaining significant help for some of his problems. It was also found that clients who are well established in life with a stable family and a good job, who have experienced relatively few problems in their lives, and who are currently faced with a sudden crisis situation appear to be much more amenable to being helped through the referral process than are the kinds of clients who are dealing with more chronic problems and whose life has a more disorganized quality.

2. INACCURATE EXPECTATIONS.—The follow-up interviews suggest that most of these referrals do not "take" because of a discrepancy between what clients expect and what they perceive the service to which they are being referred will actually give them. In some instances the difficulties seem to be related to clients' resistance to treatment, particularly if they feel that they are being labeled as having "mental" problems, since to this label there still clings a great deal of social stigma. Clients sometimes tend to feel rejected and neglected as a result of having to go through waiting periods, being referred from one agency to another, being dealt with in what they see as an impersonal or perfunctory manner, or believing that the worker to whom they are relating does not feel warmly toward them or understand them.

3. FAMILY DISORGANIZATION.—Another serious barrier to the success of the referral process is that many families are simply too disturbed and too disorganized to mobilize themselves sufficiently to get to an agency at all. In some of these cases, involving a multitude of different kinds of complex problems, the patterns of

programs and services available in different agencies are too fragmented to deal with the client effectively as a meaningful unit. In many of these instances a client's problems have to be apportioned out to two, three, or more different agencies, thus vastly complicating the referral process.

4. LACK OF SERVICES.—Often the necessary services are simply not immediately available for the client. This is particularly true for emotionally disturbed children, who are constantly faced with the long waiting lists at child guidance clinics, which are a well-known fact of life in the Boston mental health community. Other categories of patients for whom services are not readily available are adolescents, children in need of residential treatment, ambulatory psychotics, and patients discharged from mental hospitals.

5. HELPING WORKING PEOPLE.—A persistent problem, however, appears to be that most mental health and social welfare agencies do not provide effective help to low-income clients. This phenomenon has been noted in many other studies and surveys; it is probably the result of many factors—lack of congruence between agency programs and complex client needs, motivational and attitude problems, and environmental barriers. The mental health field is only now beginning to confront and grapple with these issues.

PEOPLE GIVING HELP

In this section findings will be reported that were gleaned from questionnaire inquiries directed to members of six professional groups in the community. Three of these groups were the mental health professions of psychiatry, psychology, and social work. The other three were so-called caretaking professions: those composed of nonpsychiatric physicians, lawyers, and clergymen.

Mental Health Professionals

Compared to many other parts of the country and even to many other large cities, Boston is extremely rich in its supply of mental health professionals—three or four times richer for its population than such cities as Chicago and Detroit and over ten times richer than such poorly endowed areas of the country as Mississippi. There are, for example, at least 250 psychiatrists who practice in Boston or are affiliated with Boston psychiatric agencies; there are about 120 Boston psychologists and more than double that number of social workers who are NASW [3] members —with an estimated additional 400 to 500 social workers who are not members of the national society. If to this total we add recent graduates, newer members of the professional associations, and advanced residents and students, it appears that there are up to 1,500 persons active in these three mental health professions who spend at least some of their working time in the city of Boston.

These simple quantitative comparisons of our relative wealth in professionals do not reflect certain indices of quality. We have, for example, among psychiatrists an unusually high proportion of analysts and child psychiatrists; among social workers a large number of psychiatric social workers with graduate degrees; and among psychologists a very high proportion of Ph.D.'s. Our mental health professionals are also exceptionally seasoned and experienced. The average number of years of experience in the sample studied are fifteen for psychiatrists, nine for psychologists, and twelve for social workers.

PSYCHIATRISTS.—In the patterning of Boston's mental health services the three mental health professions have distinct modal roles. The average psychiatrist spends about half his time in private practice and the other half in a psychiatric setting, where he devotes himself primarily to tasks of supervision, teaching, and training, having little direct contact with patients. He spends about 20 hours a week in private practice, carrying at any one time 10 or 12 patients. He sees between 20 and 30 new patients a year, accepting almost half of them for treatment and referring

[3] National Association of Social Workers—the social workers' professional society.

most of the others elsewhere. Psychiatrists are rarely affiliated with an agency other than a mental health facility.

PSYCHOLOGISTS.—Psychologists, too, tend to cluster in the mental health agencies, but to a lesser extent than do psychiatrists. The psychologist's role varies considerably in different types of agencies, but from an overall point of view his main function is research. Training and treatment are also activities in which large numbers of psychologists spend a good deal of their time. Even within psychiatric agencies there is a considerable variation in the psychologist's role. For example, in child psychiatry settings the psychologist spends much time in diagnostic testing and a substantial amount of time in individual psychotherapy. Almost four out of five psychologists report holding more than one job, a number of them having three or more. About one out of three does some part-time teaching, and about one out of four reports having a part-time private practice.

SOCIAL WORKERS.—Of these three types of mental health professionals, social workers are most widely distributed throughout the community in different agencies. They perform a greater variety of functions and deal with a much more heterogeneous population than do members of the other two disciplines. About one-third of the social workers sampled are employed in family service or child welfare agencies and about one-quarter are employed in psychiatric agencies. Despite the greater variety of activities engaged in by social workers, in virtually every setting their major activity is direct casework with clients. This emphasis on casework can be discerned even more clearly when data for workers are separated out from those for persons in supervisory and executive positions: caseworkers report an average of 24 hours a week devoted to direct service to clients.

Supervision and administration account for other large segments of social work time. The traditional social work emphasis on the importance of supervision is maintained in the Boston area.

The evidence indicates that at the minimum one hour of staff time is spent in supervisory activity for every three hours spent in casework.

The Allied Professions

In recent years, thinking about the care of the emotionally disturbed has tended to emphasize more and more the role of "caretaker" or "gatekeeper"—the individual in the community who is the first point of contact with the emotionally disturbed person, who identifies him, and who to some extent controls or influences his entrance into the channels of mental health services.

Although all the connotations attributed to the idea of the "caretaker" role are not fully borne out by survey data, it is clear that practitioners of all three professions that were studied—lawyers, clergy, and physicians—do come in contact with and *identify* large numbers of emotionally disturbed persons. What each does thereafter varies considerably.

LAWYERS.—Although individual lawyers identify relatively few emotionally disturbed persons among their clientele—an average of five or six per year—there are so many lawyers in Boston that their combined totals add up to 12 to 15 thousand persons. Most lawyers find that they are unable to deal with emotional problems in any meaningful way within the context of the lawyer-client relationship. In most instances, therefore, they make no attempt to do so, and in only a minority of cases is referral information provided to clients. In very few instances is any active referral process initiated.

CLERGYMEN.—The average clergyman sees in his professional capacity some fourteen or fifteen persons a year who are emotionally disturbed. In addition, of course, he is aware of emotional disturbance in many others—either in his congregation or in other persons with whom he comes in contact in his professional capacity. He refers about one out of every four persons who seek his help, almost always to a psychiatrist or a psychiatric agency.

The others he tries to help himself, through counseling and other kinds of direct assistance.

It is interesting to note that the average clergyman tries to help, through his counseling and in other ways, about the same number of disturbed persons as are accepted for treatment each year by the average psychiatrist in private practice. Since the number of practitioners in each profession is about the same—approximately 250 of each—it follows that there are about as many persons "in treatment" with Boston clergy as with Boston psychiatrists. Further, since clergy deal with persons primarily from their own congregations, while psychiatrists draw clients from all parts of metropolitan Boston, less than a third of whom are residents of the city, it also follows that clergymen provide a resource for help with emotional problems for about three times as many Bostonians as do psychiatrists in private practice.

PHYSICIANS.—Physicians other than psychiatrists, such as general practitioners, internists, and pediatricians, report with considerable uniformity that about one patient out of every five seeks medical help for symptoms that are directly indicative of emotional disturbance. This amounts to some 300 patients a year for the average physician, about three-fourths of whom he treats directly himself, relying mostly on medication but also on reassurance and supportive interviewing. Projections from the sample studied indicate that an estimated 100,000 persons a year are provided with prescriptions for tranquilizing and antidepressant drugs by Boston physicians.

While physicians refer elsewhere only a minority of their emotionally disturbed patients, the total number in this category is estimated to be about 30,000. Most of them are referred to psychiatrists or psychiatric agencies.

As a simple summary of the extremely important role played by nonpsychiatric physicians in the mental health field, it can be stated that of all emotionally disturbed persons in Boston who are provided with some kind of direct service almost two-thirds are given this service by their physicians.

IV. Places—The Agencies

The task of servicing and attempting to help the many thousands of emotionally disturbed persons in Boston is shared by a variety of different agencies. The psychiatric agencies in the city see only a small minority of Boston's emotionally disturbed residents. The remainder are taken care of in such other settings as social work agencies, correctional agencies, general hospitals, and public health nursing organizations. The information that is presented about these agencies in this section and that is summarized in Table 4 was obtained directly from about four-fifths of the city's social work and psychiatric agencies and from city departments. The roles of correctional agencies, general hospitals, and public health nursing services were inferred from interviews with several key persons in each field. Once again, caution is recommended in interpreting the specific numbers that occur in this report. The data from which these numbers were obtained are both incomplete and estimated, and therefore precision cannot be attributed to them. They are intended to provide approximations and guides as to the general order of magnitude involved.

SOCIAL WORK AGENCIES

Boston has many social work agencies—almost 75 different facilities—most of which have independent status but some of which are joined together as branches of a parent federation or agency. There are many social workers in these agencies—a total of about 500 full-time workers, of whom about three-fifths have graduate degrees in social work. These agencies service almost 100,000 persons each year. Among these are about 12,000 persons who are handicapped by emotional disturbance. Most of the latter are dealt with directly by the agencies themselves, only a minority being referred on to other resources.

TABLE 4. NUMBER OF PATIENTS SERVED AND STAFF IN SELECTED BOSTON AGENCIES.

TYPE OF FACILITY	TOTAL* NUMBER	ESTIMATED NUMBER OF PROFESSIONAL STAFF		ESTIMATED NUMBER OF CLIENTS CONTACTED		ESTIMATED PROPORTION EMOTIONALLY DISTURBED	ESTIMATED NUMBER OF EMOTIONALLY DISTURBED CLIENTS SERVED	
		FULL-TIME	PART-TIME	BOSTONIANS	OTHERS		BOSTONIANS	OTHERS
1. Social Work Agencies								
Group Work	51	200	1600	75,000	5,000	6–7%	4,000	200
Casework	22	300	60	5,500	11,000	40%	1,400	3,100
Total	73	500	1660	80,500	16,000	12%	5,400	3,300
2. Psychiatric Agencies								
Inpatient	10	—	—	4,000	1,000	All	4,000	1,000
Outpatient	13 (17) †	—	—	2,200	5,000	All	1,000	2,500
Total	18 ‡	135	275	6,200	6,000	All	5,000	3,500
3. City Agencies								
Public Schools	1	15	—	90,000	—	5–10%	Few	—
Public Assistance	1	250	—	35,000 §	—	n.a. ‖	All #	—
Total	2	265	—	125,000	—	n.a.	n.a.	—
TOTAL	93	900	1935	211,700	22,000	25–30%	over 12,000	6,800

* The number of facilities can be counted in several ways, since some agencies have more than one facility—e.g., an inpatient and an outpatient service; others retain a separate identity though part of a federated unit.
† There are 17 clinics in 13 agencies, since several agencies operate two or more different outpatient services.
‡ The total number of psychiatric facilities is only 18, since several have both outpatient and inpatient services.
§ The Boston Department of Public Welfare reports a caseload of 6,000 families and 20,000 individuals. It is estimated that this totals some 35,000 different persons.
‖ For the total caseload this figure was not obtained; within the aid-to-families-of-dependent-children program it is estimated that about half the clients are sufficiently disturbed to require intensive casework or psychiatric treatment.
Agency executives indicate a belief that staff and services are generally inadequate for the needs of most clients.

30

Casework Agencies

About one-third of Boston's social work agencies can be included in the broad category of casework agencies; the others can be considered group-work facilities. The casework agencies have a total caseload of well over 16,000 persons each year. Almost 8,000 of these are considered to be clearly emotionally disturbed, and close to 5,000 of this group are accepted for direct service by the agencies. Over 1,000 are referred elsewhere, most frequently to psychiatric resources. The great majority of both clients and workers are concentrated in ten agencies, which function as traditional family service or child welfare facilities. Six casework agencies report having 20 or more caseworkers employed. Most casework agencies make use of psychiatric and psychological consultation, although only a small number of psychiatrists and psychologists are used for this purpose. Often one psychiatrist will serve as a consultant to several different agencies.

The data indicate that casework agencies provide one of the strongest and most important links in the chain of mental health services. First of all, they serve as a collecting station to which many other agencies and individuals refer persons with emotional disturbance and through which a number of individuals are channeled to psychiatric resources. More important than their referral function, however, is their treatment function, since almost two-thirds (about 5,000 out of 8,000) of the emotionally disturbed with whom they come in contact are given direct services.

Group Work Agencies

Group work agencies can be divided into two general categories: those providing intensive contact with clients and families and an emphasis on group work, which are typified by the average settlement house; and those having more extensive contacts and greater emphasis on recreational activity, which are typified by the average YMCA. The latter agencies are more numerous and tend to attract a more representative, "normal" clientele. Their mental health role can be conceived largely as preventive work, such as social support, development of skills, and other kinds of socialization. The settlements and neighborhood centers, located for the most part in neighborhoods with high rates of social pathology, service a more vulnerable group of clients, and their membership includes a larger proportion of individuals with actual or potential emotional disorder.

The recreationally oriented agencies report that only a small proportion of their young people are emotionally disturbed—two or three per cent of the total membership. These agencies tend to have memberships of between 1,000 and 1,500; two or three supervisory staff, one or two of whom have a graduate degree; and 25 or 30 other part-time leaders and staff members. Except in a preventive sense, their mental health role is relatively minor.

On the other hand, settlements report a considerably higher proportion of emotionally disturbed persons among their members—an average of about ten per cent. These agencies have memberships of between 1,500 and 2,000 persons, with a somewhat larger staff of both full-time supervisory personnel and part-time group leaders. In these agencies we also find a higher proportion of workers with graduate degrees.

For a variety of reasons—primarily motivational factors within the clients and such situational factors as travel distance to other agencies and the endemic waiting list—emotionally disturbed clients of group work agencies are said to be very difficult to refer for more focused and definitive treatment. Therefore, settlements provide direct service to most of the disturbed persons with whom they are in contact. It is estimated that over 4,000 emotionally disturbed clients are being included in the programs of these group work agencies.

There are new developments in the neighborhood-center field through which many people are consciously striving to redefine the role of the neighborhood center in the light of new conditions. An example of these trends is the establishment of settlement outposts in public housing projects, which gives promise of the development of techniques for bringing help more effectively to disorganized families. Several persons in Boston are exploring methods of providing consultants from psychiatric agencies to help staff members of group work agencies with the many and varied mental health problems that they encounter. Preliminary work suggests that the settlement house represents an important mental health resource with some undeveloped potential. The approximated statistics mentioned above underscore this last point. Group work agencies come in contact with more emotionally disturbed children and adolescents than do the child psychiatry facilities, and they give direct service to a considerably larger number. Since these agencies have great difficulty in achieving effective referrals, and since it is unlikely that the caseloads of the child guidance clinics can be greatly expanded, these findings point to the importance of strengthening the mental health role of the group work agency.

PSYCHIATRIC AGENCIES

Boston has a large number and variety of psychiatric agencies, under both public and private auspices, employing huge numbers of mental health professionals. Many of these agencies play a key role in training mental health professionals not only for Boston but for other parts of the country and of the world. Some of these agencies are also major research centers.

Inpatient facilities range in size from the state hospital with almost 3,000 beds to small units in general hospitals with as few as a dozen beds. Outpatient clinics see as many as 1,500 new cases a year or as few as 100. Professional staffs range in size from five persons to more than a hundred. There are federal, state, and city agencies; privately supported nonprofit agencies, both independent and attached to general hospitals; and proprietary psychiatric hospitals. It is difficult, within such a range and variety of facilities, to speak of "typical" or "average" agencies. Rather, in this section an effort will be made to convey a sense of the total quantity of psychiatric resources available.

Inpatient Facilities

The major inpatient facilities are the state hospitals and Veterans Administration hospitals, which account for about 95 per cent of the beds and close to three-quarters of the admissions. The remainder of the facilities are accounted for by private hospitals and by psychiatric inpatient facilities in nonprofit general hospitals. About 4,000 Bostonians are officially hospitalized for mental illness every year, 70 per cent of them being first admissions. An additional several hundred are hospitalized unofficially, in that they are admitted to open psychiatric wards that are not categorized as licensed psychiatric institutions. Average length of stay varies markedly from one institution to another, ranging from considerably less than a month to over a year.

Many changes in mental hospital practice have occurred over the past few years, some of which had their origin or early usage in Boston. The proportion of voluntary patients has risen considerably; the development of day hospitals and night hospital services has increased; active experimentation with emergency services and alternatives to hospitalization has taken place; and the roles of all the disciplines have expanded considerably.

A major unsolved problem is provision of effective after-care services. It has been demonstrated in other parts of the country that adequate after-care services can reduce the hospital readmission rate from 45 per cent to 15 per cent. At the present time only half of the patients discharged from mental hospitals are provided with any after-care services, and these are often minimal. Organized programs for discharged patients are available in Boston, but only for a small number and, for the most part, on a demonstration basis. These range from clinical service to the half-way house and include vocational rehabilitation programs, combined social and pre-vocational rehabilitation services, and sheltered workshops. This aspect of service for the emotionally disturbed seems to be by far the weakest link in the chain and the one most in need of additional investment of time, money, and staff resources.

Turning from the exit door to the entrance door, one also notes indications, based on several local demonstration programs, that effective alternatives to hospitalization can be developed, so that large numbers—several informed observers estimate that the figure is as high as 50 to 60 per cent—of hospital admissions can be avoided. Endeavors along this line would also seem to deserve high priority.

Outpatient Facilities

The dozen outpatient clinics in Boston, divided about equally between facilities for children and for adults, have about 7,000 applications for help each year, the great majority of them from new patients. Approximately 2,000 of these applications represent children. About one-third of all applicants are Boston residents. On the average, about half of the patients who apply to a clinic are accepted, although this varies considerably from one clinic to another, ranging from a low of 30 per cent to a high of 60 per cent.

A matter of considerable concern, particularly to professionals from other agencies who deal with psychiatric facilities, is the problem of the waiting period and the waiting list. It is extremely difficult to estimate with any sense of accuracy the average waiting period between application and the beginning of treatment, or the average length of time a patient remains in treatment. Most clinics do not keep such statistics. There appears to be a general pattern in childrens' agencies of operating on a yearly cycle, with relatively long waiting periods. Almost all patients who apply and are accepted for treatment during the course of one year are assigned to treatment by the following year. The practice in clinics for adults varies more widely: some adhere closely to a policy of very short waiting periods of a week or so and no waiting list; others have long waiting periods and long waiting lists. A very rough estimate is offered that the average waiting period is in the vicinity of four to eight months.

Information on length of time in treatment is also difficult to obtain. On the basis of partial data it seems that only about half of the patients who begin psychiatric treatment continue for more than a month or two.

Long-term intensive psychotherapy is the major form of treatment offered at most clinics, although there are a number of agencies that stress, to a minor or major degree, such additional techniques as the use of group therapy, short-term treatment, and other approaches. Again basing the conclusion on partial information, the survey staff estimated that the number of patients treated each year per clinic staff member ranges between 10 and 20. The amount of time devoted to direct service of patients—including intake studies, diagnostic studies, psychological testing, and actual treatment—falls between five and ten hours per week per staff member. In evaluating this information, one must remember that the majority of psychiatric facilities in Boston devote a great proportion of their staff resources to research activities, to extensive training programs, and to various kinds of services in the community, as well as to direct service to patients.

Staff Resources

Psychiatric agencies in Boston employ over 200 psychiatrists, the majority of whom are part-time, about 60 or 70 psychologists, and over 100 social workers. The social workers are mostly full-time employees. There are, in addition, well over 200 persons in training—psychiatric residents, psychology trainees, and students of social work. Professional staff members spend most of their time in training and research activities, with clinical services being furnished primarily by those who are still in training. This generalization is most true for the psychiatrist, least true for the social worker. These figures underscore the fact that this complex of agencies constitutes one of the major mental health training and research centers in the entire country. This could not remain true if there were a radical shift in the balance of service time as against research and training time.

CITY AGENCIES

Since this Mental Health Survey was focused primarily on the city of Boston proper, particular attention was paid to the city agencies themselves. In this section two agencies that are in contact with large numbers of the emotionally disturbed are described in some detail.

The Public Schools

From among the 90,000 students in the Boston public schools over a thousand referrals a year are made to the Division of Pupil Adjustment Counseling, the major mental health resource within the school department. This division, which at the time of the survey had a small staff of about a dozen counselors, is quite limited, and its activities tend to be concentrated on diagnostic services. It is quite probable that there are many other disturbed children in the schools who are not referred to the division, and the referral patterns imply that some school principals are more interested in, and oriented toward, mental health problems than are others.

On the basis of recent prevalence studies in other large cities, it can be safely estimated that a minimum of 6,000 children in the public schools alone are handicapped by emotional disturbance. It has been recently estimated that well over 300 children in Boston are severely enough disturbed to be eligible for inclusion under the new state-aided education program for emotionally disturbed children. While substantial numbers of these children may be found among the caseloads of child guidance clinics and social agencies, the majority of them are receiving little or no help. Certainly the small, overworked staff of the Division of Pupil

Adjustment Counseling is able to contribute relatively little in the way of help for this vast number of children.

From the point of the view of the schools, the problem is lack of resources. Dr. Frederick Gillis, recently retired superintendent of the Boston Public Schools, has stated that "due to the dearth of facilities many children are deprived of therapy which has been deemed necessary by competent physicians or consulting psychiatrists."

From the community's standpoint, the outstanding fact is that the public schools' internal resources for helping emotionally disturbed children are extremely limited, probably more so than in any other large northern city. It would seem advisable that overall mental health planning for the city be aimed to some extent either at provision of more direct services within the school system itself or at development of more effective methods of channeling emotionally disturbed children to other resources for help.

The Welfare Department

The Boston Welfare Department administers the largest social service operation in the city, having at the time of this survey a total of more than 250 workers, who serve 6,000 families with children and an additional 20,000 individuals in adult programs. Although there are a few graduate social workers on the department's staff, mostly in supervisory positions, the great majority of workers do not have social work training.

The department has several assistance programs, ranging from aid to families of dependent children to old-age assistance. There is general agreement that problems of emotional disturbance and social pathology are found in greatest abundance and are of most significance among families receiving aid on behalf of their dependent children. The department has concentrated a considerable amount of its overextended resources on this program, and it is on this aspect of public assistance services that the survey focused.

Approximately one out of every 60 families in Boston is receiving aid-to-dependent-children funds. In the more disadvantaged sections of the city the concentration of AFDC [4] families is much higher. By definition, of course, almost every such family is one that has been broken either by death, divorce, separation, or desertion or is a one-parent family by virtue of illegitimate parenthood.

Extensive social and emotional pathology is evident within these families. Over one-fifth of them have one or more members institutionalized for a mental disorder or have had a member appear in court as a juvenile delinquent or as an adult criminal. Truancy and dropping out of school occur frequently, as do neglect of children and excessive drinking. Departmental staff workers believe that three out of ten of these families are in need of intensive casework services and that an additional one in five has a member in need of psychiatric services, so that at least half of these families are suffering from a degree of marked disorganization or disturbance that clearly calls for intervention.

Only a small minority of those in need of such services, of course, are receiving them. The department itself does not have the resources to supply such enormous quantities of intensive service, and other resources are not readily accessible, both because of referral problems and because of other demands on casework and psychiatric facilities.

In other cities it has been found that of all families in the community evidencing disordered behavior one-third to one-half are receiving help from public assistance sources. It is reasonable to assume that a similar pattern exists in Boston, on the one hand indicating the concentration of pathology in this element of the

---

[4] Aid to Families of Dependent Children.

population and on the other hand emphasizing the inadequacy of the resources made available to the department for dealing with these troubled people. Clearly, any shift in the distribution of mental health resources in Boston must take into account the functioning of this important agency and the extent to which additional help is required for it to deal more effectively with its clients.

OTHER AGENCIES

Because of limited resources, it was not possible for this survey to cover the complete range of agencies that are dealing with, and offering services to, the emotionally disturbed. Many additional types of facilities play a role in this pattern of service, and in this section some of them will be mentioned and briefly described.

Correctional Services

For example, the facilities of the Youth Service Board and those of the Division of Legal Medicine of the State Department of Mental Health, as well as probation and parole services, deal daily with substantial numbers of emotionally disturbed persons found in the ranks of public offenders. There is no consensus as to what this proportion actually may be. There is a tendency for *mental health professionals* who are engaged in work with this segment of the population to believe that a great majority are disturbed; on the other hand, *professional workers with a correctional orientation* are inclined to think that relatively smaller numbers are actually emotionally disturbed. It is known that almost one-fifth of persons imprisoned in state institutions are provided with some psychiatric services. Those who are engaged in providing this treatment firmly believe that it can be effective, that larger numbers would be treated if staff resources were available, and that such treatment would have a significant effect on the future careers of these public offenders.

General Hospitals

In the same way that nonpsychiatric physicians take care of large numbers of emotionally disturbed middle-class patients, the outpatient clinics of general hospitals care for thousands of emotionally disturbed lower-class patients. Clinic administrators estimate that at least a third—sometimes as many as one-half—of their patients present primarily emotional symptoms, and these persons are treated for the most part with methods similar to those used by the physician in his private practice: reassurance, support, and medication. Older patients, who tend to be very lonely and depressed, make up as much as one-third of this group.

Public Health Nurses

Another extremely important link in the mental health network is the public health nurse, of whom there are approximately 150 in the two major agencies in Boston—the Visiting Nurse Association and the City Health Department. These nurses are in contact with many thousands of patients every year, a large proportion of whose illnesses contain mental health components. A point of considerable concern to the public health nurse and to the mental hospital administrator is the actual and potential role of the nurse in assisting patients discharged from mental hospitals. Mental health consultation services are available in both nursing agencies (mostly on a demonstration basis) to aid the nurses in dealing more effectively with mental health problems in their practice, so that they will not have to rely completely on referral of these problems elsewhere.

Other Services

Other important services are those available for alcoholics, such as the clinics sponsored by the State Public Health Department's Division of Alcoholism, Washingtonian Hospital, and Alcoholics Anonymous, and voluntary alcoholism agencies. There are also several small demonstration programs in the field of vocational rehabilitation of the mentally ill that appear promising. Newly organized services for persons threatening suicide and for chronic-problem families, and similar activities that were not covered in the survey, also point the way toward new approaches to specialized types of mental health problems.

V. Summary of Findings

SOME COMPARISONS

The foregoing array of data can be related in a number of different ways. A few examples of these interrelationships can be offered as another way of picturing some of the factors in Boston's mental health scene:

—Only about half of Boston's emotionally disturbed persons receive any sort of help at all.

—Nonpsychiatric physicians provide care for about twice as many emotionally disturbed persons as do all other resources combined.

—Casework agencies treat twice as many emotionally disturbed patients as do psychiatric clinics.

—Workers in settlements, Boys' Clubs, etc., have twice as many disturbed children in their care as do child guidance clinics.

—The number of Boston children referred to the Pupil Adjustment Division of the public schools is about twice the total number of Boston children treated in child guidance clinics.

—Clergymen counsel twice as many Bostonians as are in psychotherapy with private psychiatrists.

—Within the caseload of the Department of Public Welfare alone, the number of emotionally disturbed persons in need of help exceeds the total number of patients treated in all Boston outpatient psychiatric clinics.

—The number of Bostonians advised to seek outpatient psychiatric treatment or actively referred to outpatient resources is, at the very minimum, four times as great as the total number of persons who actually apply for such help.

THE QUESTION OF VALIDITY

Throughout this first part of the survey summary the reader has been warned that the numbers used were based on estimation, not on counting. Nevertheless, it was considered necessary to report the numbers—not as facts and statistics but as indices of an order of magnitude, as a basis for such comparisons as those cited immediately above.

The questions may be asked, "What if the estimates are very inaccurate? What if the numbers are quite incorrect?" In the first place, many comparisons and checks were made of data derived from different sources, usually revealing a high degree of internal consistency. For example, in section three data were reported on the number of psychologists, psychiatrists, and social workers employed in Boston. These data were gathered from questionnaire replies submitted by several hundred individual mental health professionals. In section four, on the agencies, similar data were reported on numbers of professional personnel employed by agencies. The data from these two sources were consistent with one another.

In the second place, the numbers can be read—in context with one another—to provide a fairly good picture of the structural scheme of Boston's mental health services. Whether Boston physicians treat 40,000 or 50,000—or even only 30,000—of Boston's emotionally disturbed persons is not at this time the question of greatest moment. The major point is that the numbers are very large and, most important, that physicians are the ones providing service to the vast majority of all Bostonians receiving any service at all. Similarly, whether 1,000 or 2,000 Bostonians are receiving outpatient psychotherapy in psychiatric settings is not the major issue. The main point to be made is that the number is, both relatively and absolutely, very small.

It is for this reason, then—to try to give a picture of the total structure—that the survey findings have been so often reported with the use of such phrases as "much greater than," "only a small minority," "three or four times more than," and similar expressions.

THE STRUCTURE OF BOSTON'S MENTAL HEALTH SERVICES

Following this line of reasoning, it is possible to set forth in a very brief and condensed form some of the major structural features of Boston's network of mental health services.

1. The process of identifying, caring for, serving, and treating the huge numbers of emotionally disturbed Bostonians is a task shared by a great variety of agencies and professional persons— over 100 agencies and several thousand individual professionals. Within this vast network the most important segments from a *quantitative* point of view are nonpsychiatric physicians—first by a wide margin—followed in order by nonpsychiatric social agencies and psychiatric agencies.

2. When services are looked at from a *qualitative* point of view, however, there is widespread agreement that emotionally disturbed persons are most appropriately treated by the definitive methods used by mental health professionals in psychiatric settings. Two relatively homogeneous and small groups of disturbed persons typically receive such treatment: in outpatient settings, the young, educated, well-motivated persons with chronic character disturbances that hamper their development as productive and skilled members of society; and, in mental hospitals, the aged, the brain-damaged, the poor, the misfits, and the isolates—those whose inability to cope with life's reality, coupled with their lack of any social relationships, allows for no alternative disposition to admission to a hospital.

3. Within the mental health network the distribution of patients within the different segments is not random. Subgroups of

patients—such as those in mental hospitals, those counseled by clergymen, those treated by the family doctor—can be clearly characterized. The major dimensions of these characterizations— whether they are determinants or only correlates—are age, sex, social class, type of symptomatology, education, and place of residence.

4. The data suggest quite persuasively that the amount and quality of help that an emotionally disturbed person will receive is directly dependent on the familiar factors of income, education, color, and residence in slum or suburb. The middle-class white suburbanite with a good job and a good education has a vastly greater chance of being helped effectively than does the low-income black resident of the inner city.

5. This finding is reflected in data on the referral processes within the network, which indicate that vast numbers of persons are identified and referred for help, while only a small minority actually receive any help. The blue-collar man is least likely to be involved in a successful referral.

6. A related factor is found in the distribution of professional personnel. Highly trained and skilled professionals are clustered in agencies that are in contact with small numbers of emotionally disturbed persons, while agencies understaffed with untrained workers are attempting to deal with huge numbers of disturbed poor people, whose mental health problems are typically embedded in a complex of social, educational, and other adjustment problems.

DISCUSSION
OF THE ISSUES
❧

I. Some Stumbling Blocks

In the first part of this report, survey findings were summarized in some detail, with relatively little interpretation. In this chapter, some conclusions will be drawn from these findings, with particular emphasis on some of the obstacles that impede more efficient functioning of the total network of mental health services in Boston and suggestions for the planning of future improvements in that network. Four major topics will be considered in the first section: (1) *the grave problem of incompleted referrals;* (2) *the problems that arise from ambiguity about specific responsibilities;* (3) *personnel problems; and* (4) *problems of uneven distribution of services throughout the population.*

THE REFERRAL PROCESS

The results of this survey indicate that the process of referring for help persons with emotional disorders operates very inefficiently. Other health and welfare surveys in Boston and studies looking at the total range of social welfare services in Cleveland

46

and other cities have arrived at a similar conclusion—that referral practices in general do not work well.

A Many-Sided Problem

The findings imply that the causes of this situation are multiple and complex, and consequently a search for simple solutions should be avoided. There are, for example, problems of a technical nature having to do with the actual process of referral—a process that is basically a part of professional casework practice. Referrals carried out by untrained people are apparently not done with the same degree of technical skill as those executed by trained caseworkers—particularly those who specialize in referral. There are problems that are related to the availability of services. One outstanding example in this connection is the fact that most psychiatric clinics are extremely crowded and have waiting lists and, usually, waiting periods. Finally, there are problems related to the motivation of the client himself, and it is evident that many unsuccessful referrals reflect indecision or ambivalence on the part of the client as to whether he wishes to pursue his quest for help.

There was some indirect evidence in the survey data of a condition that has been documented and discussed in the literature reporting other research and surveys—that is, that there are special problems in providing services, including referral services, to working-class clients. It has been suggested that this is partially due to differences in values, differences in attitudes, and problems of communication that arise from class differences between client and provider of service. One can point to more obvious difficulties that are related to class factors. With the exception of settlements and neighborhood centers, most social welfare agencies tend to be centrally located and are thus geographically removed from the sections of the city where the working-class population is concentrated. This matter of sheer distance between the client and the agency can be of some concern when practical arrangements, such as for transportation or care of children, have to be made.

The "System" of Referral

But more basic than any of these factors is the question of the appropriateness of the referral model for different kinds of problems involving emotional disturbance. The manner in which people with emotional disturbances are identified and referred is based upon the traditional ways in which people with physical illnesses are identified and referred. This is a system with roots in the long tradition of medicine and public health.

(1) THE WAY THE SYSTEM WORKS.—The system assumes that a person is "sick" with a specific "disease" and that the problem to be solved is one of movement—getting the person from the point at which he is identified as sick into the hands of someone who is skilled in "curing the disease." For example, a public health screening program to identify persons with tuberculosis or diabetes follows up identification by referring tuberculous or diabetic individuals to physicians for treatment. This is an example of a clearly appropriate referral, and the system for accomplishing it is one that has worked extremely well.

(2) WHERE IT DOESN'T WORK.—On the other hand, consider the case of a depressed and defeated working-class housewife turning to someone for help with a multitude of problems that are overwhelming her: an alcoholic husband who disappears for days at a time; the piling up of pressing debts; an eviction notice from the landlord; two children in diapers and a third who is enuretic; a sickly daughter and a neglected oldest son whose school work is worsening daily; headaches and stomachaches; increasing trouble with her neighbors as she becomes more and more short-tempered; and a growing sense of guilt as she finds that she herself is turning more and more to liquor for consolation.

If this woman were to be viewed in a narrow mental health context, it is possible that she would be diagnosed as suffering from depression; and, if she were so diagnosed or identified, it is likely that she would be referred for psychiatric treatment. Possibly she would be identified as a person with marital problems and then be referred for marital counseling. The question that comes to mind is: how logical would such a narrow identification be? It is likely that this woman would not be viewed as a suitable candidate for psychotherapy; and this judgment would probably be correct, since she is neither introspective nor verbal, nor does she consider herself "mental." Most important, she would tend to perceive talking to someone once a week for a long period of time about her feelings, her thoughts, and her many worries as a totally inadequate method of helping her solve her problems.

Aside from the probable futility of referring such a client for counseling or therapy, however, one must consider the question of whether it is even appropriate to make such a referral—to abstract, as it were, a "disease" from this complex of problems. Her "depression" is a condition that might seem quite natural in view of what is happening to her. To call her situation a marital problem seems, not only to her but to most people, a rather glaring understatement.

(3) WHY IT DOESN'T WORK.—It is suggested, then, that in this woman's situation the strict application of the usual system of referral is not suitable. Her emotional disturbance, her marital difficulties, are discovered in a context of serious social disturbance and are only parts of an interlocking system of problems. It may be that these realistic problems should be considered and dealt with as they exist—that is, as a total unit, without any attempt artificially to pull out one or another of the problems for separate treatment or to squeeze a complex situation into a diagnostic mode which does not fit it.

The inefficiency of the present referral machinery in Boston has been pointed out. It seems quite probable that this inefficiency is not primarily the result of technical or administrative inadequacies, or of insufficient staff time, or of the many other factors that do, of course, play a significant part, but rather that the process itself—the traditional system of referral—is not really relevant for a large proportion of the cases to which it is applied. There is indeed a mental health component in the woman's situation, but it is only one component. She does have a psychiatric problem, but it is only one of her many problems. It may be that, if she is to receive help at all, she must receive help for her total situation.

Problems After Referral

At the other end of the referral channel, particularly if the channel leads to a psychiatric clinic or to the office of a private psychiatrist, additional problems present themselves—problems of criteria for client acceptability, such as motivation, treatability, and prognosis. As a generalization, it may be said that the patient whose life is reasonably well organized in a way that conforms to the standard American pattern, whose problems are largely internalized and tend to be unitary rather than part of a disordered social pattern involving other persons, and whose symptoms can be classified readily and converted into psychiatric diagnosis will be considered "motivated" and "treatable" and will be the most likely to gain access to effective mental health services. For other types of patients such services will be less readily accessible, and the services that they do receive will tend to be viewed as a second-best, or perhaps a fourth-best, substitute for psychiatric treatment.

Such a perception is not necessarily accurate. It can be argued persuasively that this pattern is appropriate, that the motivated, treatable person *should* have priority access to traditional methods of treatment such as intensive psychotherapy, and that change should occur not in the numbers and variety of patients for whom psychotherapy should be provided but in types of services available for broadly disorganized persons—particularly those of low-income status—with a complex of primarily social problems either overlying or growing out of intrapsychic difficulties.

Need for a Change

What is undeniable is that present referral practices constitute a serious problem. Most important, they do not work and they involve many distressed persons in a process that does not provide them with help and that doubtless leads to increased frustration and unhappiness on their part. In addition, large amounts of professional time are used in fueling this cumbersome referral machine.

THE RESPONSIBILITY PROBLEM

Closely related to the issue of separating emotional disturbance from other kinds of disturbance is the issue of responsibility for services to the emotionally disturbed. At present, this issue is shrouded in ambiguity.

The question, basically, is: In the field of services to the emotionally disturbed, who is responsible for what? Superficially, there appears to be general agreement that, ideally, all emotionally disturbed persons are properly the responsibility of trained mental health professionals. Survey findings show that practice differs markedly from this ideal state, and the temptation is strong to plunge immediately into a consideration of this discrepancy.

But another question must be given priority: What is meant by "mental health services?" The answer to this question is dependent on a shifting frame of reference. Limiting cases can easily be found: no one would urge, for example, that a psychiatrist should engage directly in public assistance work, or that a group worker should practice psychoanalysis. It is in the large area between the obvious limiting cases that ambiguity is abundant. While this ambiguity is not easily resolved, it is immediately apparent that the term "mental health services" can be considered to have at least two general and quite different meanings: (1) *all professional services directed to the emotionally disturbed that are intended to ease their distress;* and (2) *services that require psychiatric training or training in closely allied fields*—and the latter is narrowed in most persons' minds to mean psychotherapy in its various forms.

Resolving the Ambiguity

Analysis of the survey findings highlights three factors that contribute to this ambiguity about responsibility for services. First, there is the dual connotation of the term "mental health services," just discussed. Second, there is the assumption previously mentioned that somehow all emotionally disturbed persons are the responsibility of mental health professionals. This assumption rests heavily on the analogy between physical illness and mental illness and the ready, but perhaps not very well thought out, transfer of ideas and traditions about medical responsibility. This analogy, though reasonably defensible when applied to extreme states of psychosis, breaks down rapidly when it is applied to less severe states of disturbance, especially when they are manifested in behavior disorders and, most particularly, when they occur in conjunction with other kinds of social disorders. The third factor is a hidden assumption, made by many, that all persons who are handicapped by emotional disturbance are entitled to services to lessen their handicap. In practice, society has made no such commitment and there is no mechanism for providing services to all who need them or even to all who request them.

Now, if we accept the assumption that all behavior disorder and all emotional disturbance are the general province of the psychiatrist and the other mental health professionals, obviously the province remains unoccupied. At present only a beachhead has been established. Further, in view of the scarcity of mental health professionals, which will continue for many years to come, it is unlikely that the beachhead will be extended in any dramatic manner.

No one questions that psychotherapy as such should be done only by persons trained to do it. Questions that do remain unresolved are (1) what should be the role of the mental health professionals in providing other kinds of ameliorative, adjustive, or quasi-therapeutic services to the emotionally disturbed; and (2) how does one delimit the group on which the direct-treatment services of mental health professionals should be focused?

With respect to the first question, one extreme position would be that services intended to help emotionally disturbed persons should be provided only under the auspices and direct supervision of qualified mental health professionals. The position at the opposite extreme would be that no involvement of mental health personnel is necessary for the provision of such services. Intermediate positions would emphasize consultative and training roles for mental health professionals.

Positions on the second unresolved question would range from a belief that scarce mental health manpower should be reserved for treatment only of those persons with well-defined intrapsychic and interpersonal problems and who are considered motivated, "treatable," and capable of benefiting from service, to a belief that such manpower should be used for treatment of all types of disturbance in which emotional disorder plays a role.

Resolution of these questions could push the patterning of mental health services in one of two general directions, which can be briefly outlined.

MENTAL HEALTH PROFESSIONALS.—If mental health professionals are to maintain in fact the theoretical responsibility—which many assume to be theirs—for direct treatment of the total range of all emotional disorders, a major redeployment of personnel is called for. As has been pointed out, mental health professionals are largely concentrated in their own agencies, which tend to attract and deal with a specialized population. In order to encompass a vastly greater range and variety of patients not only would new methods have to be devised to reach a much larger population, but also present treatment methods and routines would have to be adapted so that much larger numbers of patients could be handled. A resolution along these lines would call for commitment to extreme and drastic changes in the present scheme of things.

NONPSYCHIATRIC AGENCIES.—But there are compelling reasons to suggest that mental health services for persons with complex patterns of social and emotional pathology—and this necessarily implies most services for persons of low socioeconomic status— may very appropriately be removed from the province of accepted psychiatric responsibility. Not only are many of these persons not well adapted to the standard psychotherapeutic procedures, but the intertwined strands of social and psychological disorder can rarely be resolved by the skill of the mental health professional alone.

If such a line of reasoning is to prevail, however, and if services for certain clearly defined subgroups in the population are to be considered the primary responsibility of nonpsychiatric agencies and individuals, it is necessary for all concerned to have a clear understanding that this is both appropriate and desirable. It is necessary also for the community to recognize the intolerable handicaps placed on certain agencies—notably those with largely untrained personnel—when, with only a fraction of the resources necessary to perform the task, they are required to deal effectively with clients who, along with all their other problems, are suffering from emotional handicaps. To carry this reasoning to its logical conclusion might, as a highly hypothetical example, induce Boston's mental health professionals as a group to forgo expansion of their own budgets and programs in favor of a drastic upgrading in services and personnel for local departments of public welfare.

Further, this kind of development would make it necessary to abandon the myth of medical responsibility and to adapt to the fact that, now and in the foreseeable future, most mental health problems involving social disorders—and probably most mental health problems of poor people—are properly and explicitly the responsibility of nonpsychiatric interests. In such a case, the primary responsibility of mental health personnel would be to provide as much consultation, supervision, training, and other kinds of direct and indirect support as possible.

The Lack of Total Coverage

One factor to be considered in looking at this question is that outpatient psychiatric service, unlike most health and welfare services, is not organized to provide total coverage responsibility by either public or private agencies. In other service areas, such as foster care, financial assistance, and hospital care, there has been a clear-cut assumption of total coverage responsibility by either a public agency or a set of private agencies. If a child is in need of foster care, and if no one else takes this responsibility, the public child welfare agency must. Similarly, no one with an acute illness in need of hospital care is permitted to do without it and no one who is destitute is permitted to starve.

In the mental health field it is, relatively speaking, only a handful of persons—the severely and blatantly psychotic—to whom this principle applies. For the great majority of the emotionally disturbed, there is on the part of the community no commitment to total coverage. This condition may also contribute to the general ambiguity about where in this field responsibility lies for providing service.

THE PERSONNEL PROBLEM

Want in the Midst of Plenty

One of the most paradoxical of Boston's mental health problems is that we have one of the highest concentrations of mental health professionals in the world, exceeded, in relation to the population, only by two or three large cities like New York. At the same time, many observers perceive a severe shortage of staff and facilities.

For example, reports of the National Institute of Mental Health provide information about professional staff resources in outpatient psychiatric facilities. Analysis of these reports for the entire Metropolitan Boston area (which is necessarily the only realistic unit for such an analysis) reveals that these resources add up to the equivalent of 270 full-time professional staff persons. In contrast to this is the presumed ideal norm for such resources—the yardstick of a clinic team for each 50,000 of the population—that has been established by the American Psychiatric Association and other groups. By this yardstick—which is generally considered a somewhat utopian ideal—our total supply should number about 200 such persons. In other words, for all of Metropolitan Boston, our supply of outpatient psychiatric resources exceeds by over one-third the number generally considered an ideal goal.

Even with this vast array of resources Boston's clinics are not able to accept more than half the patients who apply for help. At the same time, waiting periods are usually long and waiting lists proliferate, and other agencies and professionals remain understandably frustrated by their inability to make effective referrals to these facilities and to arrange for prompt care of patients in their charge.

These sobering facts raise some serious questions, first of all about the directions in which solutions should be sought to some of these problems. It seems quite unrealistic, for example, to think of increased quantities of mental health personnel as a reasonable solution, even if dramatically larger supplies of money and manpower were actually available. Further, these facts point to the need at least to examine thoughtfully the present patterns of clinical practice and the present distribution of valuable personnel.

Training and Research Responsibilities

In considering this situation, a point of great importance is that many of the large psychiatric agencies in Boston represent major training resources for psychiatrists, psychologists, and social workers. Boston's complex of training centers is one of the most important in the country and, indeed, in the world. In addition to training, large amounts of staff time are spent on research activities. Other staff time is devoted to the process of administering the various clinics and, particularly in the clinics sponsored by the State Division of Mental Hygiene, to consultation with public school systems and other agencies.

The Productivity Issue

Nevertheless, the fact remains that only 20 to 25 per cent of professional staff time is used for direct patient service, including intake, diagnostic study, and psychological testing, as well as treatment. This estimate does not take into account the time of students and residents but refers purely to the time of regular professional staff members. While the factors of research, administration, and consultation just mentioned account in large measure for the relatively small amount of direct patient service produced by outpatient psychiatric facilities, it should be noted that by no means do they account fully for this phenomenon. For example, among the many clinics of the Division of Mental Hygiene throughout the state, which devote relatively smaller amounts of the time of their staff members to training and research activities, the service output tends to be about the same as that of training clinics; in addition, fewer than one-third of the patients who apply are accepted for treatment.

Although this issue is also one of great complexity, it seems likely that energy devoted to improving the productivity of present resources would represent a worthwhile investment.

THE UNEVEN DISTRIBUTION OF SERVICES

One highly significant conclusion emerges undeniably from the findings of the survey: that for some people help is both more easily accessible and more readily used than for others. The characteristics of the "some" and of the "others" that seem most relevant are those of social class and, peculiarly, place of residence.

The Advantages of Being Middle-Class

If one assumes a dimension along which types of service can be ordered on the basis of amount of relevant training, it can be said that at one end of this dimension is the psychiatrist in private practice. Moving toward the other end of the dimension, one comes to services offered in psychiatric clinics, services offered in family service and child welfare agencies, and so on down the line. In other words, a logical case can be made that there is a hierarchy of mental health services related to the presumed skill of the practitioners involved. Accepting as valid the idea that different services can be ranked in this way, one can see rather readily that high-ranking services go to high-ranking people. The solidly established middle-class white American has a much greater chance of obtaining the skilled services of a trained and experienced mental health professional than do poor people. Having more education, being young, being female—these are additional characteristics that increase the probabilities of a given person's receiving skilled service. These links to social class are, in some measure, obvious reflections of sheer ability to pay for private care, but the same kinds of relationships, only slightly attenuated, have been observed in studying the process of selection and rejection of clients for treatment in public and low-fee clinics.

There is no evidence to suggest outright bias as a cause for this situation. It is more probable by far that the historical basis of the development of services by mental health professionals resulted in types of services adapted primarily to middle-class clients.

Nevertheless, it cannot be denied that a pattern of inequality does exist and a significant challenge remains unmet: what new developments in mental health services are required in order to make help more readily available to low-income people with emotional problems?

It is true that emotionally disturbed poor people can get their lives into a terrible tangle. It is equally true that the tangles poor people get into can make them very emotionally disturbed. In both cases, mental health workers have a professional as well as a humanitarian stake, and it is upon them that the responsibility rests to initiate solutions to the problem of maldistribution of services.

Geography

Turning briefly to the question of the factor alluded to as "place of residence," we find in the survey interesting patterns not immediately susceptible of easy interpretation. It does seem, however, that there is an interaction between the social-class factors and the environmental factors mediated by the general term "place of residence." Take, for example, the Back Bay and West Roxbury, which are sections of Boston roughly equivalent in social rank. West Roxbury has a very low admission rate to mental hospitals and appears to have virtually no patients coming to see psychiatrists in private practice. The Back Bay, on the other hand, has a somewhat higher rate of admissions to mental hospitals and has a substantial number of patients in private psychiatric treatment. Compare also Roxbury and East Boston, which are both relatively low in social rank. Roxbury shows a considerably higher rate of mental hospital admission and a slightly, but insignificantly, higher rate of patients in private psychiatric treatment.

One possible explanatory factor is the family status of these residential areas. Both the Back Bay and Roxbury have a high proportion of single and unattached individuals and of one-parent families, whereas West Roxbury and East Boston are areas in which most residents belong to regularly established families. This presumed factor of isolation and separation, which may be significant, would logically be related to rates of hospital admissions, since it is an established fact that most persons admitted to mental hospitals are not functioning members of stable families but tend to be single and unattached individuals who do not have resources that can be used as alternatives to hospitalization.

These underlying factors, particularly the factor of social class, are not ordinarily apparent in considering emotionally disturbed persons one by one. However, in view of their seeming importance in determining distribution of services, it would appear desirable that they be taken into consideration in any planning effort geared toward improving the overall distribution of mental health services in Boston.

II. Planning Urban Mental Health Services

DIFFERENCES BETWEEN "PROBLEMS" AND "NEEDS"

In this section of the survey report, additional comments will be offered as interpretations of the findings. In particular, an effort will be made to focus on the necessary linkages between problems and services and on the principles for planning that are implied by these linkages.

Planning Should Be Problem-Centered

In social planning there is a readiness to assume a one-to-one relationship between problem and need, to conclude that identification of a problem is equivalent to assessment of a need for a specific type of service. For example, the observation that in a given community there are many families in which discord between husband and wife is prevalent may lead to the assumption that the community is in need of a family service association. Alternatively, depending upon the orientation of the observer, a need might be perceived for a program of family-life education or for the establishment of a marriage counseling service. The more extreme form of this logic can be recognized in the conclusion that, because a given area has a high incidence of mental hospital admissions, it is therefore badly in need of an outpatient mental health clinic. More subtle examples can also be observed, such as the common finding that, since there are large waiting lists for services of mental health clinics, more of these clinics or more staff for existing clinics are needed.

While these observations and assessments may be valid in some ways, it should be kept in mind that repeated studies have indicated the source of bias which can creep into the too ready translation of "problem" into "need": it has been repeatedly demonstrated that an agency staff person who observes a family problem of one kind or another will very likely conclude that the family needs whatever service *his* agency has to offer, whether it be therapy, foster care, adoption, or public education.

Stated in concrete terms, the suggestion being made here is that there is a difference between asking how many new clinics (or mental health centers or hospitals) are needed in Boston and asking how many new or revised mental health services are needed *to deal most efficiently and effectively with the array of problems that actually exist.* What is being urged is that evaluation and planning be *problem-centered* rather than facility-centered or agency-centered.

The Process of Identification

In this connection, the process of identification is worth serious consideration. Persons are identified as being emotionally disturbed and in need of help by a variety of agents in many different settings. Three processes of identification may be observed: first, self-identification of intrapsychic or interpersonal difficulties; second, self-identification as a person in need of help without the perception of emotional components; and third, identification by others without self-awareness on the part of the disturbed person. Examples of these three broad categories, in order, are the person who goes to his doctor because "his nerves are shot," the person who goes to an agency because he can't hold a job and needs help in finding a new one, and the child who is identified by the classroom teacher as disruptive or troubled but who is not so perceived either by himself or by his family.

It is necessary to examine these identification processes very carefully in order to discover their implications for provision of mental health services and in order to clarify the responsibilities and appropriate functions of the multitude of agencies and individuals involved in the network of mental health services.

(1) SELF-IDENTIFICATION: THE PSYCHIATRIST'S PATIENT.—Consider the specific requirements in the extremely sophisticated process of self-identification that must take place for a given individual to become engaged in individual psychotherapy with a psychiatrist in private practice. A person must (1) identify himself as having emotional problems; (2) assume responsibility for them; (3) be willing to talk about himself and his problems; (4) have some knowledge about psychiatry and psychiatric treatment; (5) have positive feelings towards psychiatry; (6) be able to afford private treatment; and (7) embrace a value system by which he is willing to expend the substantial amount of money and time that private treatment requires. Such an identification process necessarily results in culling out an extremely specialized sample of the population.

(2) TYPES OF SELF-IDENTIFICATION.—Even within the category of self-identification as a person with emotional or "nervous" problems the varied connotations of such identification determine the point of entry into the mental health network, which in turn

determines to a large extent the additional pathways open to the patient. For example, it is extremely important whether a person labels himself in his own thinking as "sick," "troubled," "lacking," or "victimized," for the kind of service he seeks initially is determined accordingly. If he is "sick," he will probably go to a physician, which is what most people do. This is the modal form of mental health service in Boston. Physicians appear to believe it is effective, and, judging by the reports of the Joint Commission on Mental Illness and Mental Health, patients agree with them. Mental health professionals may not agree.

(3) COMMUNITY IDENTIFICATION: THE HOSPITAL PATIENT.—Admissions of persons to mental hospitals also involve complex identifications, primarily by families, physicians, the courts, and the police, but also by other agents such as neighbors and social agencies. Major factors in the process of identifying a person as a candidate for hospitalization are the extent to which the behavior resulting from his disturbance is intolerable to those around him, the extent to which his disturbed behavior is visible in the community, and whether or not he has access to alternatives to being admitted to a mental hospital. So it is that a large number of persons admitted are in no sense psychotic and a very large number of psychotics are never considered for admission.

MENTAL HEALTH NEEDS AS VIEWED BY PROFESSIONALS

Throughout the course of the survey, attempts were made by a variety of different methods to obtain the opinions of mental health professionals themselves as to the major mental health needs in Boston. In this section a listing will be offered of the outstanding problems as noted by these professionals, with brief comments relating these to other survey findings.

Inadequate Facilities

Five categories of patients are frequently mentioned as having little or no provision made for their care: discharged mental patients, working-class multi-problem families, the aged, adolescents, and children—particularly children in need of residential treatment. With regard to facilities as such—in the sense of new buildings or institutions for caring for these types of patients—only the glaring lack of residential treatment facilities for children is outstanding. It is probable that most of the services needed for other categories could be provided within existing frameworks.

Waiting Lists

Waiting lists as a major problem might be considered at first glance simply another way of talking about the need for more staff or even for a greater number of facilities. In a more important sense, it reflects some dissatisfaction with current standards of practice, which have made the waiting list an established part of clinic procedures. There is some indication, derived from comments of professionals, that waiting lists could be considerably diminished by reduction of inappropriate referrals. Other suggestions related to this problem refer to various methods of increasing the number of patients per staff member. Some agencies are experimenting in this direction with such approaches as short-term treatment and greater use of group psychotherapy.

Coordination

The need for a mental health planning body to coordinate existing services and to promote a more efficient use of available personnel is readily apparent to almost every observer.

General Social Problems

The direct relationship between social problems and mental health is not only becoming more and more clear; it is increasingly becoming a matter of concern to thoughtful persons in the field. The stressful effects of poverty, poor housing, unemployment, racial discrimination, and inadequate schools are evident in many instances of emotional disturbance. There is a great deal of sentiment in favor of mental health professionals and interested citizens taking a much more active role in dealing with these issues.

Personnel Needs

Almost every agency feels that it is understaffed. Realistically, however, there is considerable evidence that substantial increases in the numbers of mental health professionals cannot be expected. Such a forecast suggests the importance of focusing on more efficient use of present staff resources and on upgrading less-well-trained or untrained staff members in many social agencies. The need for changes and additions to deal with these problems within established training programs is also frequently mentioned in the survey responses.

Costs of Private Care

The fact that private psychiatric treatment is expensive is recognized as a reality which cannot be readily changed. Actual reductions in fees charged by psychiatrists would seem to be out of the question, since psychiatrists do not now earn as much as many other specialists. What has been suggested is experimentation with shorter treatment sessions, short-term therapy, and private group therapy. Social workers and psychologists, who do not have the traditional obligation of physicians to contribute part of their time on a voluntary or nominal salary basis, conceivably may be encouraged to increase their participation in private practice at lower fees than those charged by psychiatrists. There is also the possibility of partially subsidizing private treatment on a contract basis for patients who cannot meet the full cost from their own resources. Finally, it has been urged that the prospects of developing insurance plans to cover costs of psychiatric treatment be investigated.

SUGGESTED PRINCIPLES FOR PLANNING SERVICES

In our section on "stumbling blocks," several of the general overriding mental health problems in Boston were discussed—referral, responsibility, personnel, and distribution-of-service. In this section the difference between problems and needs has been pointed out and some of the specific problems and needs perceived by professionals have been mentioned.

Some General Issues

In relation to ways of meeting the problems identified, three general issues emerged from the findings and comments: centralization, specialization of function, and the relationship between program and need.

(1) CENTRALIZATION VS. DECENTRALIZATION.—Centralization of services doubtless makes for greater efficiency and improved administrative control. On the other hand it must be recognized that among the emotionally disturbed—particularly those from the working class and those with widespread life disorganization —there are realistic and motivational problems which limit mobility. Ideally, services for these people should be close at hand in their own neighborhoods. In planning for improved mental health services for Boston, then, we must first consider whether a particular service or agency should be more centralized or decentralized in relation to the types of persons it is intended to help.

(2) SPECIALIZATION VS. MULTIPLE FUNCTION.—Regarding specialization, there appear to be a fair number of agencies in Boston whose functions partly overlay. The survey findings suggest a need to consider what might be the ideal range of agencies, with respect to how many and what kinds of special-function agencies there should be and what kinds of programs could be joined together in different multiple-function agencies.

For example, should all the child welfare agencies take equal responsibility for treating emotionally disturbed children, or would it be more efficient for one or two of them to take this specialized responsibility? How many different child guidance agencies and outpatient child psychiatric clinics are needed? How many different outpatient psychiatric clinics for adults are needed? Are there logical ways in which some of them can specialize, as the independent child guidance clinics have specialized with respect to age of patients? Can similar specializations be worked out with respect to research and training, as against direct service to clients? This question must be considered in context with the issue of centralization. For example, it seems logical that there should be a large number of decentralized settlement houses in Boston but a relatively small number of centralized psychiatric agencies offering traditional psychotherapy.

(3) PROGRAMMING FOR NEED.—A final significant issue to be discussed is that of programming with as much regard as possible for actual need. Specifically, in considering what quantity of new mental health services is needed in Boston, community planners should be prepared to think about such questions as:

(a) For provision of additional child guidance services, would it be logical to expand largely in centralized centers, perhaps with formal attachment to existing private child guidance clinics and outpatient services?

(b) For provision of a broader range of community mental health services, such as crisis intervention, preventive activities, and consultation, what are the logical units of decentralization?

(c) For provision of supportive and consultative services—and perhaps in-service training and direct services—for other types of social agencies, what is the appropriate administrative arrangement?

A Hypothetical Example

It is possible to conceive of a public program with three major types of facilities: a small number of centralized intensive-treatment centers, a larger number of perhaps six or eight community mental health centers in different neighborhoods of Boston, and an additional agency service facility which could provide supportive services directly to other agencies on a city-wide or even a metropolitan basis. This pattern is suggested merely as an example of the kind of planning that may emerge when the proposed principles are applied to the problems as they now exist.

III. Needed: A Problem-Solving Mechanism

WHAT IS MISSING

While the findings of the survey reveal a situation in Boston in which the overall pattern of mental health services is fragmented and inefficient and reflects poor distribution, they emphatically do not reveal or imply the intention on the part of any agency or profession to initiate or maintain such a situation. The problem does not reflect arrogance, willfulness, or indifference on the part of the many highly skilled and hard-working professionals who are dealing with Boston's emotionally disturbed population. What is missing, rather, are established channels of communication and existing platforms upon which these professionals may meet and plan together. In the absence of such formal mechanisms it is idle to expect coordination simply to happen spontaneously. Clearly, what is needed is a stable problem-solving mechanism, through which all of the relevant agencies and professions in the city can work together toward improving services. Staff evaluation of the findings of this survey indicate conclusively that the number-one missing link, the outstanding need, is an on-going mental health planning body for Boston.

HOW IT MIGHT BE DONE

An important point to be made here is that mental health problems are the concern of a great variety of both public and private agencies and that basic philosophical decisions overlap into the provinces of universities and of professional societies. A major requirement for a planning body is that it include significant representation from, and possibly financial support by, all relevant bodies—i.e., psychiatric agencies, social agencies, city and state departments, universities, and the professional societies, added to the nucleus of the three sponsoring agencies for this survey (the Division of Mental Hygiene of the Massachusetts Department of Mental Health, the Massachusetts Association for Mental Health, and United Community Services).

There are several different forms which such a planning body could take. It could be established as a permanent part of the existing planning machinery. It could begin its life as a special planning project. It could be attached for administrative purposes to the existing planning agency or the existing voluntary mental health association or to one of the state agencies. It could exist as a newly created independent body.

In whatever form the planning body would be most acceptable and feasible, it seems undeniable that new machinery for formal planning in the field of mental health is an absolute necessity. It is probable that only through such a body can the necessary steps for rational change be taken.

APPENDIX

※

RESEARCH METHODOLOGY
USED IN THE SURVEY

The preceding summary report was based on one-and-a-half years of investigation and a large number of specific findings. In this appendix section a more detailed presentation will be given of the methodology used, together with a discussion of the scope and limitations of the Boston Mental Health Survey.

The design of the survey was shaped both by the breadth of the questions being asked and by the severe limitations of time and staff resources. The survey period was predetermined as eighteen months and the staff resources consisted of a half-time director and three part-time associates. The conscious decision to look at the broadest possible range of activities affecting the emotionally disturbed established an additional limitation as to the intensity of the fact-finding operations: it was necessary to rely largely on secondhand sources purveying estimated information. In addition, data were often based on a sample from a poorly defined population and the exactness of projected findings was therefore questionable.

Sources of Data

There were four major sources of data: inquiries to agencies, inquiries to individual professionals, published reports, and a follow-up study of a cohort of patients who had used two community information-and-referral services.

Sixty-five mental health and social welfare agencies provided information about their caseload and staffing patterns, with particular emphasis on the proportion of clients handicapped by emotional disturbance and the types of service or referrals provided to these clients. These agencies provided this information either through questionnaires filled out by agency executives or, in a few instances, through interviews with survey staff members.

Questionnaires were sent to six groups of professionals: psychologists, psychiatrists, social workers, physicians, lawyers and clergymen. Over 600 questionnaires were returned—an overall effective reply of almost 40 per cent.

The questionnaires to the mental health professionals asked for information on such points as place of employment, approximate proportion of time devoted to different functions, and opinions about mental health problems in the Boston area. Questionnaires to the other professionals focused on number and proportion of emotionally disturbed persons seen in individual practice, referral patterns, services offered, and perceptions of mental health needs. Psychiatrists, physicians, lawyers, and clergy were all asked to provide individual case studies.

A study of specific referral practices involved a follow-up investigation of 140 emotionally disturbed patients who had applied for help consecutively to the Red Feather Information and Referral Service [1] and to the referral service of the Massachusetts Association for Mental Health during September, October, and November of 1960. In this study an inquiry was made of the agencies to which the individual clients were referred and then, at a point approximately one year after the initial application, personal interviews were conducted by the survey staff with a sample of 20 of the clients themselves.

[1] This service is conducted by United Community Services of Metropolitan Boston.

Three hundred and forty case studies were gathered, of which 241 were complete and the remainder were incomplete in one respect or another. These included 65 full studies and 90 additional short studies from psychiatrists, 28 from lawyers, 41 from physicians, 51 from clergymen, and 65 from group work agencies.

In addition to collection of the specific data described above, extensive use was made of existing reports, census data, annual reports from agencies, studies done by the Department of Mental Health and other agencies, and similar documentary material.

Finally, it should be pointed out that a good deal of background information was obtained by interviews and small group meetings with more than 100 agency executives, staff members, and community leaders.

Methodological Problems

COLLECTION OF CASE STUDIES

One of the methodological problems that presented considerable difficulty in interpretation had to do with the representativeness of the sample of case studies. The studies were obtained, for the most part, by asking each respondent to furnish a single case description, including the client's residence, age, family status, presenting problem, and disposition.

The clergy, lawyers, and physicians were asked to report on their most recent case involving emotional disturbance. These instructions, however, were not followed uniformly, a fact that was indicated by obvious references in the questionnaire returns to time considerably in the past.

Instructions to psychiatrists were more precise, in that they suggested a method for randomization, either on the basis of a time factor or on the basis of a rule for choosing a random case from closed files. Inspection indicated that these instructions were followed closely by almost all respondents. The sample of cases from psychiatrists indicated an unusual pattern of residential distribution, which seemed to warrant additional investigation. Therefore, a second request was sent to a sample of psychiatrists asking them to report age, sex, approximate street address, and disposition, regarding their three most recent patients. This procedure provided an additional 90 short case studies. Case studies from group work agencies were assembled through the agencies themselves, with individual staff members being requested to furnish one current case description involving emotional disturbance.

Among all reporting respondents, despite careful instructions that they should use only Boston residents, there was apparent misunderstanding as to the actual city limits of Boston, and a fairly large number of suburbanites were accordingly included; these had to be eliminated in analyzing the residential distribution within the city of Boston itself.

QUESTIONNAIRE RETURNS

The return rates for the questionnaires from various individual professionals tended to be satisfactorily high. The specific rates were: for psychiatrists—40 per cent; psychologists—78 per cent; social workers—42 per cent; clergymen—29 per cent; lawyers— 28 per cent; and physicians—30 per cent. The total number of completed questionnaires returned for each professional category were: psychiatrists—127; psychologists—111; social workers— 118; clergymen—71; lawyers—52; and physicians—123: a final total of 602.

THE REFERRAL STUDY

The referral study cohort consisted of 101 cases from the Information and Referral Service of United Community Services and 39 cases from the Massachusetts Association for Mental Health. The 101 United Community Services cases were selected from a total of 382 cases handled by the agency during a three-month period. Those persons selected for study had obvious mental health problems observable in the brief descriptions available. Among the remaining 281 cases in the three-month sample, there may also have been mental health problems which were not so obvious or unequivocally evident.

The study proceeded in two steps. A questionnaire was sent to the agency to which the client had been referred, requesting such data as nature of problems, nature and duration of agency contact, disposition, etc. One hundred and twenty of these questionnaires were sent out, with a return rate of 93 per cent. The second stage of the study involved direct interviews with selected clients one year after their initial inquiry at the agency. Contacts were attempted with 49 clients, but only 20 were actually interviewed. In 11 cases it was not possible to find the client at home and in 18 cases the family had moved. Interviews were semistructured, lasting on the average from one to two hours, and covered the contact with the referral agency, the presenting problem, and subsequent developments.

SUMMARY

The following final summation of the data on which this report was based can be offered:

(1) information collected about agency functions and operations from 65 mental health and social welfare facilities;

(2) questionnaires filled out by over 600 individual professionals;

(3) 340 individual case studies analyzed;

(4) a follow-up study undertaken of 140 emotionally disturbed persons referred for help;

(5) unstructured interviews conducted with over 100 knowledgeable community leaders and agency executives and staff members; and

(6) a miscellany of annual reports, minutes, census data, and existing studies reviewed.

From all of these basic data the overall picture of mental health activity in Boston was derived. It can be seen that, on the one hand, the base from which the findings were derived is broad, varied, and extensive; on the other hand, it must be recognized that the accuracy of the sampling is not known and the projections that were made to the total population may not be completely accurate. In addition, it should be pointed out once more that the data themselves are not the result of direct observation but rather consist for the most part of estimates made by secondary sources.

COMMENTS ON THE SUMMARY REPORT

EVEOLEEN N. REXFORD

This survey of the mental health needs of Boston citizens—how these are being met and not met—provides us with a foundation for planning more effective ways of using our resources, the development of new patterns of service, or, indeed, totally new services. Dr. Ryan and his associates are to be congratulated on the extent of their data collection within the limitations of time and of funds available to them. Dr. Ryan's thoughtful discussion of the findings challenges our community to comprehensive planning and to further fact-finding. His description of the categories of persons with whom his survey was concerned makes it possible for each reader to understand more readily the dimensions of the problem and the importance to our city of more satisfactory solutions for the psychosocial difficulties of a large number of our citizens.

The actual fact-finding process was necessarily limited, as Dr. Ryan points out. One fact which illustrates the urgent need for a central coordinating structure within the Boston area is that comparable and meaningful data from the various agencies, institutions, and persons serving the emotionally disturbed population in our city do not exist. Only of late years, for instance, have the child psychiatric clinics, both public and private, begun to collect comparable data regarding their work, which, in turn, are shared with the National Institute of Mental Health. We have no mechanism for integrating these data with those of the casework agencies, protective services, correctional services, schools, and others also providing care and assistance to emotionally disturbed children.

The firm recommendation of the survey for the establishment of a Boston mental health board is clearly a prerequisite for obtaining a detailed picture of the present situation and for planning remedial actions. However, coordinating and planning activities on the part of such a board can be effective only if both the many professional persons directly concerned and the citizens' groups taking responsibility for the community become strongly persuaded that we must obtain more facts, plan with vision, and take action which is strongly supported beyond the period of crisis recognition.

The report of Dr. Ryan's survey must of necessity take on a global, yet selective, character. Because of the importance of this document to the area in which I have worked for many years, I should like to emphasize a few points.

1. The methods most highly evolved and most often used by psychiatrists and social workers—psychotherapy and casework —were developed for the treatment of neurotic difficulties, for persons preoccupied by inner emotional conflicts. These patients could communicate their thoughts and feelings verbally; they could come to respect and value the possibility and need for change within themselves. They have been largely intelligent people, usually educated and often middle- or upper-class in status. They might well complain of financial or social problems, but the awareness of inner emotional turmoil was never far from the surface.

During the past several decades psychiatrists and social workers have applied their accustomed professional methods to persons with more complex and perhaps more disorganizing emotional disorders, though often with less awareness of inner conflict, and to people from different life circumstances. They found that their ways of working with neurotic patients were often not effective and that quite considerable changes in methods were required to give these different groups of patients help. An important question which has not yet been satisfactorily answered is whether these groups of more refractory patients require a different application of the accustomed psychiatric methods or whether they profit more from assistance from persons with a different type of training and professional experience. In some instances, pioneers have worked out effective methods for groups once thought beyond the scope of psychiatric or casework treatment.

I want to underline that these modifications, wherever effective, have required special studies, experimentation, and tolerance for many failures. In Boston today, there are several significant research studies under way, which Dr. Ryan could not describe, directed at groups heretofore refractory to the best-known psychiatric and casework methods—in some instances, groups with a certain kind of emotional difficulty and, in others, groups from socioeconomic sectors seldom reached by our office or clinic practices.

We have had many experiences during the last half century to teach us that changing the locale of practice of psychiatrists or social workers does not solve the emotional problems of severely disorganized or disadvantaged families, nor does bringing all persons with any type of emotional disorder to such a professional individual result in their cure. We need to know far more about the make-up and the way of life of the patients we do not ordinarily see; and, having learned their needs and how they can accept help, we have to find out more about how to help them. These imperatives call for research on the part of many, experimentation in methodology, and coordination of the efforts of persons with different types of training. Such programs are going on: they require money, time, and patient support, because the participants are trying to find answers which are not known today; all we can say thus far is that they are not easily come by.

2. Closely related to the difficulties in helping certain individuals outlined above is an area we are just beginning to explore—namely, the attitudes toward help. This issue is important beyond the area of mental health services; it is crucial to programs of public health and medical care and probably to all programs for human betterment. Public health officials are asking today with a sense of urgency: "Why is it that parents do not bring their children for polio vaccine when a bus will transport them from their front door to the health unit?" Urban redevelopment officials are making public their puzzlement over why persons living in miserable surroundings do not seem to want to take advantage of new housing available to them. Settlement-house workers have long asked why families in their neighborhood who clearly could profit from their programs do not send their children and why the parents do not come to the events for adults. We are told repeatedly today of families whose members suffer from crippling emotional disorders who do not come to available facilities or do not return after they have brought themselves for one visit.

The assumption has been made by many serious professional and lay leaders that a larger number of service facilities is the answer. On the other hand, certain professional persons in Boston interpreted this survey's findings about referral failures as evidence of the inferior quality of the staff at the referral centers, just as students of medical care have often concluded that the patterns of care in certain clinics must clearly be defective if patients do not return regularly. They have not asked: "What of the patients themselves?"

There are a few systematic studies suggesting both that, until we know more of the attitudes toward help of large segments of our population, we will be sorely handicapped in providing them with the help they need and that often the community's concept of the help they need may be far from their own. If we do not develop sophistication in this area, we will continue to meet with disappointing failures and to ascribe these failures to an inadequate number of services or to faulty professional techniques.

3. In this period of increasing recognition of the mental health problems of the disadvantaged sector of our population, we are properly directing our attention to services for them. But may it not be short-sighted to deplore the use of services by the better-educated, middle- and upper-class segments of our community? Emotional disturbance is no respecter of persons, class, or status. Does our society not require emotionally healthy leaders in neighborhoods, schools, business, and government? Would it be sound social planning, even if we could effect it, to allocate all of our mental health service to disadvantaged, deprived, and blatantly disordered individuals?

The survey findings indicated that a high percentage of Boston residents receiving psychotherapy lived in the Back Bay; they were further characterized as being, in the main, single and educated. It is quite likely that many of these patients are college and graduate students, persons preparing themselves for some type of leadership in their neighborhoods and communities. We might well do our image of the total mental health needs of our society a considerable disservice if we seem to infer that only the disadvantaged and seriously ill need or deserve mental health aids.

We are properly working toward methods and patterns of service for all our population. The obstacles appear staggering, but solutions are likely to lie not in the direction of robbing Peter to pay Paul but rather in improving our existing modes, developing new patterns, and bringing a number of helping groups into more effective cooperation with one another.

4. It was one of the merits of the Report of the Joint Commission on Mental Health and Illness that its authors drove directly to the point of the large expenditure in money, time, and effort that will be needed to meet the mental health problems of our

country. They spoke frankly of the necessity for extensive research and for training of personnel. We should be no less frank in this report to the citizens of Boston.

Further, we can be certain that to deal effectively with our own mental health problems not one or two professional groups and their supporters but the whole network of helping agencies, institutions, and their supporters in both the public and the private sectors, the colleges, universities, and churches will have to put into operation a rigorous process of self-scrutiny and integration. This process, under the leadership of a mental health board, will disrupt familiar patterns, disturb vested interests, and force all of us to reach into unaccustomed areas of thinking and acting. Programs of social action will aid us greatly in our work, but the helping resources of the community must bring themselves into alignment with the psychosocial needs of our time and be prepared to reexamine, re-plan, and re-do our activities as often as the rapidly changing nature of our society forces us to keep pace.

5. The indirect contributions of more adequate mental health services to a community should be stressed. Dr. Ryan's discussion of emotional disturbance speaks to the loss which society incurs from the obvious interference with the individual's functioning. The direct return from services which restore the emotionally disturbed person to productivity, the child to progress in school, the alcoholic to sobriety is readily discerned.

However, what is often not considered is the effect upon others of the troubled individual's improvement, the indirect return to the community upon its investment. Although a child's problem brings the family to a child psychiatric clinic, the effective treatment of the child may rebound beneficially upon the whole family, the marital relationship, and the upbringing of the other children, as well as upon the management of the referred child. The man who has sought treatment for his emotional distress may deal far more effectively and understandingly with his subordinates in his office or plant. Just as one individual's psychological difficulties can create strain for others at home, in the office, or in the neighborhood, so can his more mature and settled adaptation affect those around him favorably: chain reactions can go both ways.

6. Although the cost for adequate mental health care may well seem staggering, it is important to realize that the benefits incurred for the present population from treatment and rehabilitation will make possible a healthier development adaptation and greater productivity. Financial support for such services can therefore rightly be regarded as serving an additional cause— namely, that of prevention.

II
COMMENTARIES
ON THE
BOSTON REPORT

DISTRESS IN THE CITY—AND IN THE MENTAL HEALTH FIELD[1]

※

DANIEL J. LEVINSON
Yale University

It is a truism to say that the mental health field has been in a state of flux for the past 20 years and that this condition is not likely to abate in the near future. So rapid is the change, indeed, that many current leaders who played a major part in instituting the reforms of the 1950's now find themselves regarded as "conservatives," impeding the progress of the 1960's. There is continuing and often bitter controversy in every area of work: specific therapeutic techniques, the use of partial hospitalization, the roles and responsibilities of the various professions and of nonprofessionals, the conception of "mental illness" versus numerous other conceptions of the problems and needs of those who receive our services.

Beyond the specific issues of theory and practice there is a broader and in some respects more fundamental question: *Will mental health professionals and institutions accept the responsibility for appraising and redefining the structure of the mental health field and its place in society?* This is truly a vexing question. Until recently the answer has been largely "no." Clinicians generally lack the social perspective that would provide a

[1] The writing of this essay was supported in part by Grant MH-25, 264 from the National Institute of Mental Health.

framework for raising and seeking to answer this question. Hospitals, clinics, and agencies ordinarily have all they can do to take care of current business. Professional schools and training programs tend to function as guilds, transmitting the expertise of the previous generation and being cautious about breaking new ground or questioning the institutional fabric within which they operate.

Over the past decade the picture has been changing. New questions are being asked about the health needs of our society. Health services are coming to be regarded, like education, as a right rather than a privilege. It is becoming increasingly evident that mental health services are organized inefficiently and distributed inequitably. New efforts are being made—thus far with only limited success—to assess community needs and to plan more rationally the organization and delivery of health services.

We are late in recognizing the extent of our problems and deficiencies, and the task of catching up is burdensome. At the same time, we have tremendous opportunities for social contribution and for personal-professional development. In particular, there is a need and an opportunity for the generation of multidisciplinary theory and research. The great potential of the field of community mental health is that it will contribute both to the provision of needed services and to the advancement of the science of man.

The Boston Mental Health Survey is a major contribution to the development of this new field. It provides a descriptive overview of the current state of mental health affairs (circa 1962) in a large urban center. And, what is even more important, it raises some of the fundamental issues that now confront us in our efforts to develop a more excellent, integrated, and equitable system of services for the entire society.

As Ryan indicates, Boston is one of our most affluent cities in its supply of mental health professionals. It is extremely wealthy in comparison to rural areas and is considerably better off than other urban centers, such as Chicago and Detroit. The problems and deficiencies of Boston are thus magnified many times over on the national scene. Mental health services in Boston are provided by over a hundred agencies and several thousand professionals. The facilities form a loose network; there is virtually no overall planning or integration, and the relationships between facilities are characterized more by insulation and rivalry than by collaborative effort.

The depth and magnitude of the problem are evident even in the gross descriptive findings. Ryan estimates—conservatively, I believe—that only about half of the emotionally disturbed population of Boston receives any sort of help. Of those receiving help, a relatively small proportion are seen by psychiatrists and other mental health professionals. Far larger numbers are in the care of nonpsychiatric physicians, clergymen, the Department of Public Welfare, and the like. Of the total number referred to psychiatric outpatient services not more than one-fourth actually apply for such help, and of these only about one-fourth enter some form of treatment. It is clear that a person's referral and treatment career depend less on the nature of his psychiatric problems than on his education, occupation, residential area, age, race, family support, and social isolation. It is primarily these latter characteristics that differentiate the clienteles of the state mental hospital, the private hospital, the general practitioner, the clergy, the casework agency, and the psychiatric clinic.

The various findings, taken singly, will hardly surprise anyone familiar with the growing literature on social, economic, and organizational factors in the operation of health and welfare services. The total pattern of findings, however, casts new light on the "distress in the city" and brings into focus some of the crucial sources of difficulty that must be overcome. One of the major contributions of the Ryan report is its analysis in the second section (pp. 46–69) [2] of the complex issues at the core of our problems. The issues are, in my opinion, of basic importance not only for Boston but for all parts of the country and for all groups and organizations that have a responsible part to play in improving mental health services.

I would like to comment briefly on a few of the issues raised by Ryan. My aim in doing so is not to offer easy answers but rather to suggest directions for further analysis and for exploration of new approaches.

I. Boundary Processes: Problems of Referral and Entry in Mental Health Facilities

A major goal in the provision of mental health care for the community is that *appropriate services be available to individuals as the need arises.* Even in a city like Boston, however, this goal is far from realization. This is due in part to shortages of money, staff, and resources. It is due even more to faults in the organization and functioning of the facilities and the total service network. Every facility has a variety of means, formal and informal, by which prospective patients are selectively referred to it and are then selectively screened for admission as patients or clients. Not all persons-in-need within the community are *referred* to a given facility; not all who are referred actually *apply* to it for service; and not all who apply for help are *offered* it. In most facilities the attrition rate from one step to the next is extremely high. The number of persons actually offered service is only a small proportion of the total number of persons in the community who are suffering considerable psychological disturbance or impairment.

These findings—well documented by the Boston survey and by other studies—call attention to the relation of the clinical facility

[2] In Part Two all page references to the Summary Report are enclosed in parentheses immediately following the textual reference or quotation.

to the surrounding community. They point to the need for closer scrutiny of the *boundary processes* by which a facility controls the entry of patients into its operation. By and large, the boundary processes of the facility serve to restrict severely the size and the psychosocial composition of its clientele. These processes are rarely acknowledged in official policy statements and their consequences are rarely examined by staff.

One means by which an organization exerts control over the inflow of patients is its *intake* system. In most psychiatric outpatient clinics, for example, only 20 to 25 per cent of the applicants enter some form of definitive treatment. The prospective patient's chances of gaining admission to a clinic are thus hardly better than the prospective student's chances of gaining admission to most colleges. The high attrition rate is not due to staff judgment that most applicants are in good mental health. The one thing any applicant can count on is that he will be diagnosed as having some form of mental illness.

A detailed consideration of the reasons for the high attrition rate is beyond the scope of this brief essay. I shall mention only three of them. (1) In most clinics, the main purpose of the intake-diagnostic procedures is to select "good" patients for psychotherapy and for the education of students. Applicants who do not want psychotherapy or who are judged poor candidates for it are not likely to survive the selection process. (2) Much of the staff time in clinics is spent on intake procedures, diagnostic conferences, and other screening devices—on work with applicants who "terminate" after two or three clinic visits. This creates great pressure on staff and leaves relatively little time for therapeutic involvement with patients. (3) A good deal of reciprocal mistrust exists between applicants and staff. There are few unreluctant seekers of help, especially of psychiatric help. In most applicants the personal suffering and the wish for help are counterbalanced by various opposing forces: fears of the psychiatrist; fears of actually being "crazy" and of being stigmatized by others as "crazy"; coercive pressures, direct or indirect, exerted by family, employer, or social authorities; preference for certain kinds of help and aversion to other treatment modalities. Clinicians (like teachers and others who offer highly personalized service to clients) prefer patients who are "motivated"—who acknowledge that they need help, who will accept treatment and work responsibly at it on the therapist's terms. Clinicians tend to be on guard against "poorly motivated" applicants. Thus, the reciprocal mistrust between applicant and clinician is a crucial issue in their encounter. The clinician has a major responsibility for confronting this issue, for providing a variety of treatment alternatives, and for negotiating a therapeutic contract to which he and the applicant can be jointly committed.

The selective screening of applicants is, however, only one of the boundary processes controlling the provision of services by mental health facilities. We must also ask: Who are the applicants? How is the applicant population "selected" from the much larger population of persons-in-need within the total community? These questions lead to the fundamental problem of the *referral* system—the diverse means, formal and informal, by which persons with problems are selectively referred into the mental health service network and, frequently, are shunted about from one facility to another until they either receive help or drop out. As the Ryan report shows, at least half of the population suffering from emotional disturbance never enters the mental health network. The outpatient clinics and psychiatrists in private practice have a small, highly restricted clientele. Even in state-supported clinics, where fees are graded by income, the poor, non-white, less educated, and more severely impaired are rarely referred and even more rarely offered treatment. Referral of patients from one facility to another is handled in a relatively inefficient and irresponsible manner. The goal and spirit of referral are more to get rid of a troublesome case than to provide needed help. Most facilities have no sense of responsibility for the patients they refer elsewhere and no system of follow-up to make sure that the referral was successful. Large numbers of prospective patients get lost in the lacunae between facilities. Moreover, most facilities manage not to obtain data on this important problem; the excellent referral study carried out by the Boston survey is one of the few systematic efforts made thus far to illuminate this process.

In short, the unreadiness to examine and face up to the problems of referral and intake is one of the major failures of the mental health system as a whole. The sources of this failure are manifold: rivalries between agencies and disciplines; deficiencies of leadership; inadequate understanding of mental health as a community problem; and commitment to short-term professional and organizational vested interest rather than to meeting societal needs. It is high time that these problems be confronted.

II. Responsibility—By Whom and For What?

As the Ryan report makes abundantly clear, mental health professionals provide direct clinical service for a relatively small minority of the total population of persons suffering from significant emotional disturbance. By "mental health professionals" I mean psychiatrists, clinical psychologists, psychiatric social workers, psychiatric nurses, and others who have received specialized training in this field. Their primary work sites include mental hospitals, outpatient clinics, mental health centers, psychiatric social work agencies, and private offices. Far larger numbers of persons in need receive services from other practitioners and organizations: nonpsychiatric physicians, clergymen, public welfare agencies, the schools, police and correctional systems, and the like.

At the present time, then, it is a myth to say that mental health professionals have accepted responsibility for the mental health problems of our society. The professionals who make this claim have blinded themselves to the marked constriction of our roles and to the encapsulation of our clinical facilities. In our professional work and especially in our training programs we have cut ourselves off from the life problems of all but a few segments of the population.

In recent years the picture has been changing with the emergence of the broad and still rather amorphous field of community mental health. A variety of new organizations, programs, and roles are in process of development. Since my own experience is chiefly with a mental health center, I shall take this as an example. The basic issues are, I believe, relevant to other contexts as well.

The radical new departure in the idea of the community mental health center is its commitment to take responsibility, in concert with other community groups and agencies, for assessing and dealing with the major mental health problems of a defined catchment area. An organization may, of course, be called a mental health center without fully accepting and implementing this commitment. What responsibilities should a mental health center undertake, and what services should it provide?

The forms of service that are in greatest supply and that are least problematic within the culture and social structure of the established psychiatric organization are the direct clinical services given to patients within the walls of the clinical facility. These compose the *intramural clinical program* of the mental health center. They include diagnostic evaluation, referral, and various kinds of individual and group treatment organized within outpatient clinics and inpatient units.

If the mental health center is to meet its community responsibilities, however, it needs also to develop an *extramural program.* That is to say, staff must move outside the boundaries of the center; they must regard the community as a locus of, and a partner in, mental health work. This is not an easy step. It requires a major change in traditional roles, values, and organizational patterns. The extramural activities that are perhaps least difficult to establish—that are most congruent with the traditional clinical roles—involve the provision of direct and indirect clinical services within the community. The *direct clinical services* include home treatment units, half-way houses, field stations (including "store-front" clinics), and other facilities offering various forms of patient care. The prototype of *indirect clinical service* is consultation by clinics with other community agencies (notably in education, welfare, and correction) regarding the mental health aspects of their work. The consultation is usually case-oriented, focusing on individual clients with severe emotional problems; it may also contribute to in-service training or to the development of new programs and policies. The common theme, however, is that the consultant uses his clinical skills not directly with patients but with the staff of another agency.

The newest and most controversial component of the extramural program is that which involves the staff in *social action directed toward institutional change in the community*. These efforts are not "clinical" in the usual sense; they are not directly concerned with the diagnosis and treatment of illness, although they may lead in time to the delivery of more adequate clinical services for currently disadvantaged sectors of the community. The primary aim of this work is preventive. It attempts to modify the features of the social, economic, and institutional environment that are inimical to mental health—that breed alienation, apathy, regression, and powerlessness of the individual to affect his own destiny. The mental health worker functions as a social change agent, facilitating the efforts of community groups to define their own problems and goals and to work more effectively toward improving their lot.

The role of clinician-healer is vital to society; it has been validated by history, law, and custom. The clinician endangers some of his most precious rights when he becomes more directly involved in the struggle for social change. He feels on safer and more familiar ground when he tries to change the individual patient within the professional context of his office or hospital than when he tries to change the social environment through his intervention in situations of social conflict. Not all mental health professionals can or should devote themselves primarily to the problems of prevention and social change. It is essential, however, that prevention be accepted as one legitimate function of the mental health center and as one legitimate component of the professional role. The mental health field has enormous and as yet unmet responsibilities. We must do something to change our own "establishment"—a disorganized, archaic system that discriminates massively against the most disadvantaged sectors of the population. We have a responsible part to play in other areas as well: in the improvement of the educational system, in the struggle for civil rights, in governmental programs concerning poverty, urban development, and the like.

Two caveats are in order. The first concerns our knowledge and skill; the second, our authority. As mental health professionals move from the clinical facility to the wider social scene, it is evident that our present understanding is at best limited. We have some (modest) expertise with regard to individual personality, psychopathology, and interpersonal relations. Our theoretical and practical horizons need to be broadened to include an understanding of groups, institutions, communities, and society as a whole, including its political and economic aspects. In extending our community involvement, then, we have as much to learn as to teach, and we properly enter the field as collaborators in a joint venture rather than as experts offering wisdom but gaining little in return. This new role requires a change in the traditional professional-client relationship. The professional is accustomed to being regarded as an authority, albeit a beneficent one. His authority has a somewhat rational base in his special competence and a less rational base in the fantasy (often shared by himself and the client) of his omniscience. The authority of the physician is the chief source of the placebo effect that has been the single greatest "curative" influence in the history of medicine. However, this use of authority is a serious obstacle to work in community mental health. Our effectiveness depends in large part upon our readiness to share the authority for collective effort both with our colleagues and with our clients. As each discipline comes to modulate its demand for total control over its "professional turf," we shall hopefully learn to use appropriate authority in the service of *shared responsibility* for the mental health needs of society.

III. Manpower: Problems of Training and Deployment

There is an acute shortage of trained manpower in mental health, and the prospects for the foreseeable future are poor indeed. The numbers of professionally trained psychiatrists, clinical psychologists, psychiatric social workers, and nurses are utterly inadequate for the need. Since a drastic increase in the number and size of professional schools is not likely, the problem will have to be solved in other ways. It is clearly necessary to draw upon less trained personnel, such as volunteers, "indigenous nonprofessionals," college students, and other groups. My interest here is not in the steps that should be taken to develop nonprofessional manpower. Rather, I shall consider briefly some implications of the manpower shortage for the mental health professions.

First, it is the responsibility of the professions themselves (through their societies and educational institutions) to acknowledge, understand, and deal with the overall manpower problem. This may be self-evident; but in fact the several professions have until recently devoted themselves almost exclusively to the training and care of their own members and to protecting their own vested interests against the real or imagined onslaughts of the others. In these quasi-military struggles the interests of patients and the needs of society have been given, one might say, less than full consideration.

Recognition of the manpower shortage carries major implications for professional training. I shall take psychiatric training as an example, but the problems of the related professions are similar. Residency programs in university training facilities have been oriented primarily toward preparation for private clinical practice. The first year of the residency is ordinarily spent in a mental hospital or other inpatient setting. The primary emphasis is on the resident's clinical work with individual patients. The program usually gives much less attention to his learning about the nature and the therapeutic relevance of the milieu, about the importance of collaborative relationships within the "treatment team," about the character of the hospital as a therapeutic organization, and about the relation between hospital and community. The enormous potential for learning about social and community psychiatry remains largely untapped in most first-year training programs.

The resident usually spends his second year in an outpatient clinic, where an effort is made to provide him with "good teaching cases" that will advance his understanding of psychopathology and his psychotherapeutic skills. The main function of this training is to prepare the resident for private practice with neurotic, middle class patients. By and large, the most valued part of the second-year experience is the opportunity to engage in intensive psychotherapy with a few carefully selected cases. This is often a rewarding experience, but it creates a number of serious problems. A basic distinction is drawn between the "good cases," deemed suitable for intensive psychotherapy, and the others, who are in effect "bad cases"—though they may be identified euphemistically as "unmotivated" or "poor prognosis for psychotherapy"—and for whom the resident learns to feel little therapeutic responsibility. In dealing with prospective patients, his primary goal is to determine which ones are most suitable for the major technology (psychotherapy) he has to offer. Unfortunately, the "bad" cases far outnumber the "good." In addition, many other kinds of learning potentially available in the outpatient setting are ignored by most training programs. The resident learns too little about alternative clinical strategies: brief crisis intervention, home visits, use of nonprofessionals, and the like. Beyond his work with individual patients, the resident could acquire a broader social perspective regarding the goals, structure, and operation of the clinic as an organization rooted in the community. He would then better understand the advantages and the limitations of the existing model of care. He might also develop a greater sense of responsibility for individual patients, for the improvement of clinical services, and for dealing with the mental health problems of the community.

It is often argued that the field of social and community psychiatry is a specialty, and that training in it should be one of several options electively offered only after the initial two or three years of "basic" clinical training. I would agree that such intensive work at an advanced level is desirable on an elective basis; but I believe, as indicated above, that it is essential to include a social orientation as an aspect of the initial two-year program. Otherwise, most residents go on to private practice with almost no social perspective; and those who move into community psychiatry are likely to feel alienated from the others. If the current split between "clinical" and "community" work is to be resolved, the problem must be confronted at the start of professional learning and identity-formation. This is a crucial issue for the senior staff; it requires a change from the traditional training system, autocratic in structure and monolithic in ideology, to one that is more pluralistic, flexible, and innovative.

I shall note one final implication of the manpower shortage—namely, the need for redeployment of professional staff. Most of the graduates of university training programs in psychiatry and related fields tend to remain in urban centers, working in university-affiliated clinical facilities and/or in private practice. Ways must be found to deploy professionals in more diverse geographical areas and in more diverse institutions and roles. This means, in part, that professionals must join with others in creating new work settings in which challenging tasks can be undertaken under reasonably favorable conditions. Even more, it means that many professionals must be ready to leave the clinician's office (be it in hospital, clinic, or private practice) and take on part-time or full-time roles in other institutions and community contexts. They will then devote themselves in part to clinical work with patients and to the clinical training of students. They will also participate in efforts at change in the social environment, seeking on a larger scale to prevent psychological impairment and to foster the development of the person.

To conclude: I have indicated some of the problems that must be confronted by the mental health field if it is to alleviate its current distress and contribute more fully to the needs of society. I have focused on three major issues: the boundary processes that control the flow of patients into and among mental health facilities; the problem of responsibility—of whom and for what; and the training and deployment of manpower. We can deal with these and many other issues only by broadening our theoretical perspectives and modes of work. To raise the effectiveness of mental health centers and related organizations, we shall have to understand better, and to involve ourselves in, problems of organizational structure, authority, division of labor, and the like. To develop community-based programs, we shall have to move more than ever before into the community and to apprehend its cultural, political, economic, and institutional aspects along with the psychological aspects. To improve the entire network of mental health services, we must reduce the encapsulation of the single facilities and engage in imaginative planning at local, regional, and national levels.

THE MYTHIC
AND
THE MYTHICAL

MICHAEL AMRINE
American Psychological Association

The doctor remains a mythic figure. We no longer ascribe magical powers to the astrologer or to the witch doctor. Even our modern alchemists have lost some of their aura; many of them are still interested in converting their science into gold, but they are themselves in the crucible, where society tries to turn *them* into gold. But the medical doctor still has a Faustian presence. Today, when the doctor can give us a new kidney or a new heart, we still project onto him our need for, and our belief in, magical powers for help in desperate situations. If a Kennedy's brain is blasted, or if we ourselves are told, "your X-ray indicates we had better make another lab test" we look into the doctor's face sometimes with irrational fear and irrational hope. We regard the doctor with an awe in which superstition is mixed with what we can remember about science. The doctor may not repair the irreparable, our inner reason tells us. But still he voices the decision— yes, no, or maybe the situation is not irreparable. So, in spite of everything the AMA has done to make him all too human in our eyes, and despite the fact he no longer carries a black bag or makes house calls, the doctor, like Abraham Lincoln or The Hangman, still walks in the midnights of our dreams. Possessed of scientific knowledge, practiced in art, radiant with mercy, the mythic figure of the doctor stands alone in our workaday world, having knowledge and power related to life and death.

Only an impudent questioner, armed with the cold light of scientific survey methods, would dare to ask, as William Ryan has asked, just where are the real doctors when real people have real troubles, now, today, in Boston?

In this essay we cannot examine how the "doctor of the mind" came to join all the other doctors of fact and myth. Recently many have noted that the development of psychotherapy as a "medical" province is historical, which is to say "accidental" rather than logical. Any poet would argue that for a mind diseased, as Shakespeare said in Macbeth, there has to be a doctor, and a strange one. The doctor family already has such "cousins" as Dr. Faustus, Dr. Frankenstein, Dr. Carrel, Dr. Caligari, Dr. Schweitzer, Dr. Spock, and Dr. Salk. "Naturally" this is the locale in which to produce or to place such figures as Dr. Freud, Dr. Menninger, Dr. Timothy Leary, Dr. Joyce Brothers, and Dr. Kenneth B. Clark. It will surely be agreed that all of these latter names are "names to conjure with," and that is what we are talking about—conjuring . . . expert remedies for desperate situations.

Now, turning away from myths and magic and coming to comment on mental health and William Ryan's superb finding of facts, we ask—and Ryan goes far to tell us—"What is The Doctor really doing for the psyche?" It is here that we may find that Ryan has performed an almost unique service. He has virtually shown that The Doctor who specializes in the "mentally ill" is all but nonexistent in Boston, so far as most prospective "patients" are concerned. Ryan has confirmed what only a few can face and hardly anyone can say: in the mental health field The Doctor is not only mythic, he is mythical. It is not only that we—and perhaps sometimes he—have explicitly and implicitly exaggerated his powers. It is that we—and he—have been led, partly because of the older omnipresent myth of the omnipresent doctor, to exaggerate his prevalence—that is, his existence.

Hundreds of thousands of babies are born in the U. S. each year without any physician's help—but we all believe that when anyone has a baby the doctor is called. In mental health the mythicality is similar, but even more surprising, once one looks at the simplest figures.

There has grown up in the generations since Freud what we can now see as a durable but fantastic faith: people believe that special doctors treat the emotionally disturbed. But in fact it has always been true that psychotherapy by trained specialists has never been available to more than a handful of persons. Persons with emotional disorders number in the millions. Psychiatrists and clinical psychologists number in the thousands—perhaps 30,000 to see and treat perhaps three million a year who *might* benefit from their ministrations. So the psychotherapist is all but unfindable by those who need him. These facts on manpower come closer to human understanding when they are seen in the local community and examined with precision, as they were examined by Ryan and his colleagues. It seems to me a main point is that nearly everyone wants to believe there is such a thing as psychotherapy but very few persons have seen or experienced any of it.

My own thought is that only in the age of mass media, particularly of television, could so many people ever have believed there were so many psychotherapists when in reality there are so few. There are some occupations that are intrinsically dramatic, and psychotherapy is one of them. There are others: there are many more fictional detectives than there are real detectives; and perhaps a hundredfold more men are killed on television in a week than are killed in actuality in America in that length of time. Most of us have never seen detectives but we all "know what they look like." The cinema and television have made visual a number of these dramatic occupations, which we *recognize*—but never have seen. Among them are test pilot, hangman, commander of a U-boat, and lieutenant in the foreign legion. Alongside that latter lieutenant I would put the dramatic figure of the psychotherapist, dramatized by Freud, Scott Fitzgerald, Tennessee Williams, and a thousand other men of genius or talent. I say the psychotherapist is more appealing than the foreign legionnaire. In fact, he is magnificent, but he is not medicine. He is myth.

To repeat, I am not concerned in developing this particular line of thought, nor is Ryan concerned in his study, with the truth or falsity of the psychotherapy dogmas. I am remarking that there are a million teachers in the U. S. and nearly a million nurses—they exist. But 30,000 psychotherapists are really a trace element in the population, and only a fraction of this trace are doing psychoanalysis. Regarding psychiatrists in the U. S. and their patients, only two per cent of all patient-hours are spent in psychoanalysis. Thus I say psychotherapy exists a little—but psychoanalysts are about as mighty an army as Trotskyists. The evidence indicates that psychoanalysts are more influential in Boston than are Trotskyists, but not because they actually change more individuals' lives in any deep way. Eveoleen Rexford, a psychoanalyst and an M.D., speaks in her comments on this report of "adapting" to social change; but at the same time she speaks in defense of "treating" only a few upper middle class persons, and she asks whether we are to think only of treatment for the underprivileged, since most of the persons getting treatment in Boston are destined to be leaders in the community and we need sane leaders, and so on. It seems to me Dr. Rexford has missed the point or begged the question: psychoanalysts can either center on "treating" the individual or join with some of those brother psychiatrists who speak a vague mystical "mush" about giving their skills to the whole community. To society it does not matter much what nine per cent of the active 20,000 psychiatrists do—which figure (20,000) is less than ten per cent of the number of M.D.'s, which in turn is ten per cent of the population engaged in health services. It would only matter what these 1,800 analysts did if they dispensed real medicine—pills and liquids, or some other discrete treatment which demonstrably changed the course of demonstrable illness. Forty trained surgeons, I am saying, are a lot; but 40 or 400 psychotherapists are not much for the great distresses of the city. There just are not enough psychotherapists, much less psychoanalysts, to do anything about the vast social problems of which they have begun vaguely to speak.

I once attended a meeting of Latvians-in-exile in Washington, D. C. These Latvians meet in a fine old mansion: it is ordinarily the headquarters of the United Daughters of the Confederacy. It was sad to listen to their laments about Latvian freedom and to hear of past glories while eating their incredibly good pastry in that home of The Lost Cause, under the eyes of the portraits of Stonewall Jackson and Jeb Stuart. I mention this experience here again to emphasize the problem of numbers: there are more Confederate Daughters in the U. S. than there are psychotherapists, and there are far more American Latvian patriots than there are psychoanalysts. History, in my opinion, is going to give freedom back to Latvia *and restore the Confederacy* before it is going to establish any semblance of reality to some of the psychotherapists' more grandiose claims of ability to "treat society" and even to illuminate and to "treat" the social ills which are dividing and perhaps destroying this country. Ryan shows what a small portion of the disordered really find treatment.

The whole myth of the omnipresent psychotherapist could never have bloomed except in America, where progress is the state religion. There never before has been a society of such affluence, mass media, and myth-making potential that it could make a nonexistent helper an almost tangible figure to millions of persons—in Harlem, in Appalachia, in Detroit, in Chicago's Hyde

Park, in San Francisco's Nob Hill, in Palo Alto, and in Watts. In all those places the deprived and disordered can frequently see on television quite moving and appealing pictures of psychologists and psychiatrists. At the same time in the same country only an affluent society could *keep invisible* to most psychologists and psychiatrists the vast needy populations of Boston, Harlem, Washington, Chicago, Newark, Detroit, Birmingham, San Francisco, and Watts.

The same scarcity of the central figure but pervasiveness of a myth is, of course, found to a degree in general medicine. *It is true that many persons in Harlem close to the poverty level have never seen any doctor other than Dr. Kildare or Dr. Ben Casey.* We know this absolutely in reference to prenatal and postnatal care. We know how our infant mortality rate could be lowered if we could see that every infant born in New York City had a physician to guide it. We know that most mothers in Harlem have seen that cliché movie scene in which the doctor comes in to attend the pregnant mother and immediately orders someone to boil water. *We know that hundreds of thousands of those mothers have never seen any real obstetrician, much less any pediatrician.* This is part of the mythology of American health care being the best in the world. It is the best—on television.

On the national scale we know that the reality of numbers in general medical practice starts with facts like these: there are some 300,000 physicians, if we count every last osteopath; and there are about three million persons in health services. The latter (auxiliary, ancillary paramedical, or "other" personnel) have multiplied quite considerably as modern science has developed "good things" which can be done to keep people alive. The news spreads and people demand that the "good things" be done to them and their families. The number of persons in health services is still increasing at a brisk rate, as it has been for 30 years, whereas the relation of the physician to the general population has been remarkably static.

Many interesting things have happened in general medicine (one of them is Medicare) because of these basic numbers—because science has advanced, and the supporting personnel and the demand for treatment have increased, much faster than the basic supply of core professionals. One of these interesting developments is that in many segments of informed American opinion the physician, while retaining a mythic quality, is no longer seen as God's Vice President. In fact, he is sometimes seen as the Devil's Vice President.

It is only fair to say, however, that students of public opinion find that the respect and disrespect in which the occupation of physician is held produce an image full of baffling contradictions. For example, pollsters find that some people are quite well aware of policies of the AMA; some even feel that physicians, individually, are money-hungry, status-driven, and narrowly professional to the point of unionism. People tell pollsters that doctors are capable of splitting fees and failing to live up to their ideal of humanity. The same person who expresses views much like these, however, when asked about his own personal physician, will say that he himself has found a very good doctor and these criticisms do not apply to his own doctor. It seems that the patient deifies the man he sees at the shortest range. The distant doctors—in their AMA stronghold—are evil. The one who cuts our child's throat and brings the child back alive with his tonsils gone—that man holds the keys to life and death and we will hear or say no ill of him.

There can be no doubt that a doctor takes on great mythic qualities of humanity and omniscience in the eyes of the patient who needs him most. Or we might be kinder to all—including the patient—to say that when a patient and physician have known each other for years they understand one another much better than the average newspaper reader can understand the AMA—or than the AMA leaders can understand the average newspaper reader. In any case, science keeps bringing in "good things," and more and more persons are required to dispense them. And America now turns to its health priorities and tries to look at them with the knowledge that this nation, you and I, must pay for what we get. What can we get? What should we pay?

In mental health our answers are hard to come by. In mental health we have a situation in which science is not "bringing in good things" each year nor in each five years. We are demanding them. But we are not getting them. Millions need help. Science does not answer. Psychiatry and psychology are not bringing in yearly harvests of specific remedies, cures, or palliatives for known and describable disease entities. Neither is science bringing in known preventive measures which, if followed, would absolutely reduce the number of persons who usually would come to be called—or miscalled—the mentally ill. Dr. Rexford in her codicil speaks of prevention, as many in the mental health field do, as if preventive measures were known and demonstrated.

But in fact Dr. Rexford and her colleagues really know next to nothing about *preventing* mental illness.

So, in what is called the mental health field it seems to me that, as in the general health field, there are some crises ahead with respect to the position of The Doctor. In my belief, the mental health field is overdue a drastic review of its concepts and its explicit and implicit promises. It may turn out that psychotherapists using the illness-and-treatment model will find themselves subject to successively more critical examinations by various public investigative agencies. There will be more and more agencies which will "monitor performance" in some way: there is now a wide range of agencies looking over the therapist's couch—hospital boards, insurance statisticians, union officials, federal inspectors, and state and federal legislative inquirers.

What can be done for emotional disorders? Are they really diseases? If so, are there enough physicians working on them? Are they getting results? Are services distributed according to need? Who should pay—and how—for these "treatments" if the "patient" cannot pay? How can those who pay be assured that they are getting their money's worth? Congressmen and insurance men have started to ask these questions.

But even more deadly than the gimlet eye of the insurance actuary is the mocking laughter of today's youth. The "now" generation can actually suffer life and survive, believing that not only God but also Freud is dead. The real inner core of true believers in psychotherapy, which was once so proud of being avant-garde, has suffered the fate of those gallant, forward-looking airmen who once fought the battleship admirals and who are now fighting the missilemen who look on manned aircraft as old-fashioned for their purposes.

It happens that not only is there distress in the city, there is social disaster in the city. We will need all our knowledge and all our heart to prevail—and even, perhaps, to survive. Some of the young people have, in fact, turned back to mysticism or magic. But the really sharp ones, looking at the distress in the city, are asking questions for which the dogmatic answers from Vienna of 1910 or Topeka of 1925 do not suffice.

The young people—and the refugees from disaster—are asking what the science of psychology can do now. What does the doctor of philosophy or the doctor of medicine know which can really help people as they are now?

In terms of the numbers and what can really be done I believe that the aging, once avant-garde figure of the classical psychotherapist has all the gallantry of Chiang Kai-shek. If it were not for certain powerful allies which enfold them for historical and accidental reasons, both of these gallant figures would be unprotected. Once unprotected, they would vanish into thin air.

Then we could get on with the real problems, such as what in the world to do with the individual human disasters now occurring in the grand social disaster we call Boston.

PSYCHIATRY AND THE URBAN POOR

※

LEONARD J. DUHL [1]

University of California, Berkeley

The summary report by Dr. William Ryan of the Boston Mental Health Survey presents the critical need of our urban areas for better mental health services. Its discussion of the health needs of the Boston area centers upon a population all too often ignored in our concept of urban blight—the tens of thousands of people handicapped in their struggle for life and happiness by many kinds of mental or emotional disturbance.

The most important achievement of the report is that it begins to connect the problems of mental health to the overall problems of the city. In describing the problems and concerns of the alienated sector of our urban population, which is all too often neglected in the rush for physical renewal, statistically favorable job placement, and improved transportation systems, it links psychiatry to the future of our cities.

It was this connection between psychiatry and the city that was responsible for my being in the Department of Housing and Urban Development (HUD) as a psychiatrist. I have been con-

[1] Professor of Public Health and Urban Social Policy; former Special Assistant to the Secretary, Department of Housing and Urban Development.

cerned for a long time with problems that I think are central to psychiatry but which are now central to the problems of the city as well. These are the problems and concerns of the alienated urban population.

It is no accident that psychiatrists were once known as "alienists," for they have been dealing with the problems of the alienated for a long time. The mentally ill have, until relatively recently, always been locked away. They have been hidden, put in places where they could not bother the general population; and psychiatrists have been hired to keep them from "annoying" the rest of the population.

Only gradually did we begin to open the doors of the hospitals and to realize that there was something of all of us in every patient. We began better to understand the behavior of people. Patients who formerly would have been hospitalized began filling community institutions for the mentally ill and putting pressure on community facilities at large.

Now I find that I am concerned with a broader segment of the United States. My patients are no longer the mentally ill alone but the poor in the central cities and the Negroes, who in a way have been in effect just as much locked into institutions as were the mentally ill 50 to 100 years ago. They are locked in ghettos and in public housing projects. They are locked into unemployment or underemployment and into the apathy of their run-down neighborhoods.

One of the first things I did when I moved into the Department of Housing and Urban Development was to spend my time exploring the department and how it operates. I found out fairly quickly that it is concerned with more facets of urban life that affect the lives of every one of us than any other federal agency in the United States government. It concerns itself with construction, with financing, with mortgaging, with transportation, with sewers and water, and, indirectly, with almost everything else that has to do with the city around us. And it is close to the cities' sources of finance and the big decisions that affect all of our lives.

Almost the first thing the department staff told me was that I must not really disrupt their system, because they had to be sure of a dollar returned on every dollar invested. So I started wandering around the cities to see what they were like and how this world looked to the alienated. I took helicopter rides, where I could see instantly that the city is two elements—smog and cars. The whole city is a big parking lot when you look at it from the air. Then you dip down and begin to see more. One nice thing about little helicopters is that they can go very low. You see sections of towns completely isolated; you see sections of towns where there are no buses going. From up in the air you see the buses going back and forth through all the best sections of town but not in the poor sections.

When I started wandering in this world of the alien, one of the first things I did was to go into one of the two or three (but one stands out) big public housing projects in Chicago. When someone asked me what I saw, I said, "I saw, as I looked over the public mental hospitals, a very interesting thing." And it took me a while to realize that I had said "public mental hospitals" when I was talking about the public housing projects.

I went through all of the mental illness "factories." And I found parallels to almost everything we've learned about how a hospital is run—about how a hospital, no matter how good the individual therapy is, controls and affects the behavior of the people who are in it in such a way that they get "locked in" more tightly by the institution than they are by their own pathologies and their own problems. When you get out to see some of these big city institutions, you find that the rules and regulations and procedures and the way people live in them are of the same variety that we know in mental hospitals and in the prisons and jails. The local community is an "institution" with a psychological wall around it. Culturally you cannot get out of it—you are "locked in."

And you begin to see how the apparent pathology of the ghetto is created by the welfare rules and regulations, which say that if you want to get paid for the number of dependent children in your house you had better not have a man living in it, for if one is there, you will not get paid. And so you begin to learn a technique of living without a man in the house—in other words, you learn how to "work the system."

And the people living in the institutions known as public housing know how to work the system for all it's worth. They know how to squeeze every dollar out of the organizations and the institutions available to help them, how to grab through the poverty program, and how to stay on welfare. And they do it.

I found that I had to go back to these cities because I had to ask a question. How many of these things known as cities and the slums (here I'm not concerned just with the housing projects; I'm talking about all the alienated people in the city) are created by all that we're doing in the name of cure? For example, we put up these public housing projects supposedly to cure people. Supposedly the people in them were poor people and needed better housing because they were living in dismal places. But building the housing projects is like putting up a beautiful, brand new mental hospital but not changing any of our attitudes toward its inmates at all. Very quickly the hospital gets destroyed; and, similarly, the housing project gets destroyed, while the culture—the way of life that led to its being built—remains as it was.

Some interesting things have happened this last year. I have found that we cannot divorce our concern for the alienated from our concern about what's taking place in the wide world around us, especially in the world of the poor and disenfranchised. Something very important is beginning to happen. The "system" is being confronted. And it is being confronted for very interesting reasons. The mass media and the communications people at the operational level have begun to crack down on the system. As a result, people in the inner-cities want many things to be different. They want what everybody else has. And they want to break down the walls of the institutions known as ghettos.

And they also want power. As one man told me in the middle of the slums, "I want a piece of the action, man; I want a piece of the action." They begin to press and they want to control. Another man said to me, "It's very nice in the city." It happened to be a city that gets more federal money than any other city in the United States. He said, "It's a real nice thing that this man gives all these nice things to us. He gives us big houses and big parking lots and big everything; he runs magnificent programs and he gets his name in the newspapers and magazines. But he's giving it to us, man, he's giving it to us! Paternalism is dead, doc. He can't give it to us anymore. We've got to get it and we've got to get it and rise up ourselves."

This raises a very interesting question about the alienated, which is related to my own profession. One of the diseases of the alienated is apathy. And one of the things we know about apathy is that we can't do very much about it by doing nice things for people. We can try and in doing so be more humane. We can make the living experiences of the alienated better in terms of cleanliness and health and air. But the basic disease has to be cured, has to be dealt with, in the people themselves as they begin to pull themselves out by their own bootstraps; and this they are beginning to do—first in the name of civil rights and then in what we are seeing as black militancy.

What we are witnessing is people who are tired of destroying themselves, as they have for so long, through living in slums in which everybody ignores the ones who destroy themselves. These people are now beginning to put pressure on "the system." And now we are concerned because they are opting out. When they destroy themselves we have no problem, but when they start destroying us they become a problem. They are beginning to stretch their arms and muscles to try to do something for themselves.

And we are finding fascinating developments: somewhat obscured by the black militancy today are people who are beginning to create something that looks like a resurgence of the American capitalism of the 1870's. Everybody wants a business of his own. They want to start stores. One man in the paper said, "I want to start a little store called the People's Black Market because the People's Market next door is charging me $5.00 in interest for every $10.00 I buy every week." And a black militant group in Harlem, composed of one thousand men, recently got together and started a little investment trust for themselves.

This movement reminds me of the adolescents among our own children. We see children beginning to stretch their muscles, to opt out, if you will, to rock "the system" and push on it and tell us what is wrong with it. This is a process which hurts us badly. But in the process of suppressing this militancy we very well may kill what is underneath it, which is our children's ability to grow.

The reason I am using this analogy is that I have a very, very strong feeling that if I go around the country looking at the problems of the alienated I will see too many people—people who have "made it"—completely unaware of the problems involved. This is an area in which psychiatrists can assist people in attaining understanding. We understand, and I think we have a great ability to contribute to bettering our lives, given certain caveats, which I will discuss later.

The people I have discussed the matter with have had conflicting ideas about the complex processes which might best bring about change in the community. Give the alienated better schools and better buildings, change the income tax, have a negative income tax—these ideas are widespread. All of them are pretty good. In fact, the only trouble with them is that they involve changes in our institutions and the way we do business in and through them which will take years. They involve changes in people themselves.

Think for a minute of how most of our immigrant cultures have taken three generations to become a real part of the United States. But the majority of the Negroes and many of the Mexican-Americans have remained in that first-generation status for the last 400 years. And now that they are beginning to stretch their muscles we are expecting them to accomplish everything in one generation which would normally take 40 or 50 years. And I think we can be encouraged, because they have learned some of the skills of the game. But at the same time we are going to have to change our institutions and conduct our business with more equity, more humaneness, and less paternalism and control.

HUD, previously HHFA (Housing and Home Finance Agency), for example, has allowed cities to do urban renewal. City administrations have torn down the central cities and built up nice big offices, stores, and businesses. In the process they have displaced Negroes. The Negroes call it "Negro removal." The cities blame the department for a bad tax base. What the department finally had to do about two months ago was to say that no city in the United States could do urban renewal any more unless they provided localized housing for the people that renewal would displace. This sounds like a very simple requirement. But it is rocking all urban renewal departments in the United States, because their plans are geared to building universities, holding businesses, etc., without thought of whose homes such construction may displace or where the displaced may be relocated.

Some may be aware that the riots in Newark were precipitated by the fact that urban renewal was going to displace 26,000 Negroes, so that a college of medicine could be built. And the blacks of Newark pointed out that if the college of medicine was built it was going to be taken apart brick by brick unless somebody figured out a way to deal with the problem of over 26,000 displaced people.

I am concerned about change and that we psychiatrists apply some of our knowledge of its processes to the problems of the city and of the alienated. But before we do, I think we have to deal with the question of whether we have changed ourselves. I suggest that, although we are ahead of most people in terms of understanding the processes of change, the dynamics involved, how to go about it, and the processes of resistance, we do not really know what makes the city work. We have not learned our anatomy yet. We have not learned the basic physiology of the city.

But this is not the disease of psychiatrists alone. I am quite convinced now that there is nobody who really understands how fantastically complex this living organism known as a city is. We all must begin to learn about it.

What my suggestion has been for a long time is that the only way one begins to learn about the city is the way we began to learn medicine in our internship. We used the hospital as the laboratory for learning the techniques of medicine. That new laboratory was in itself as complex as a city. And in the hospital we learned not only how a patient behaves, what diseases and illnesses there are, and what physiology is; but, if one happened to be the department chairman of psychiatry, he had to learn how to work for peace among the medical students, how to get a certain amount of time to teach, and how to negotiate.

Similarly, we have to start learning things about the city by beginning with total immersion. We've got to get in it, to see it and smell it and feel it. I am always distraught when I think that, although a city is nothing without people, in many cities people are "scared to death." Many are scared to walk into Harlem; they are scared even in cities like New Haven. There are only 30,000 Negroes and no Black Power in New Haven, but many whites have been afraid to go in with me and see the streets around which the riots took place because there were some "characters" hanging around with black turtleneck sweaters and guns hanging out of their pockets. They thought our heads were going to be knocked in. And yet we could walk in and we could talk and communicate.

The city is made up of a thousand micro-cities. And if you are trying to learn the whole of the city and how it operates as a total organism, you have to find out what each micro-city is and how all the pieces and parts fit together.

How do you learn about it? I don't expect all of us to become experts on the city. I certainly do not know in detail how to run a city, and I never want to be a mayor or city manager or the like. But we have to learn what the problems are. How does the mayor operate? When people build big new towns, what are the problems of financing? We psychiatrists get called into cities, old and new, and must learn as much about them as possible.

Incidentally, the psychiatrists of Johns Hopkins University became involved in setting up a psychiatric program for a brand new city of 120,000, called Columbia, located between Baltimore and Washington. But before they could do anything they had to learn about how this city operated. They had to learn one cardinal principle: the man who was building the city wanted to make a profit. This profit motive applies to all cities. No matter what we want to set up, we must first learn the language of profit and loss.

If we psychiatrists are to learn something about a mayor, we must first learn what power is, because some of the things the mayor stands for require that people give up power generally or equally. He asks decision-makers to shift values; he asks them to shift the way they think about things, to have more concern with people's needs. We must know about the mayor's values and concerns. We must observe the mayor and how he operates and how his budget is operated. We must see how his transportation system is run and how he makes decisions regarding it.

Somebody may say, "Well, why worry about transportation systems?" If you are a psychiatrist, you worry because that is how your patients get to you. The transportation system links up the city. I have rarely seen doctors that demanded better transportation for their city, and yet it is essential to their practice.

I suggest that we know very little about the city. Something very strange, very interesting is happening in the confrontation existing between "haves" and "have-nots" in the city. The pressure is being felt by every professional; the lawyers feel it, the city planners feel it, the people in public administration feel it. Almost everyone I meet in the universities feels the pressures of social change.

What I propose is that, instead of moving into the laboratory of community psychiatry, we use the entire community as a laboratory. And though there are some things that we as psychiatrists have to learn by ourselves, there are many others that we can learn together in joint curriculums and joint programs. We should learn together not only because it is easier but because we must learn each other's language so we can talk the same game.

Working at HUD, I think the hardest problem I had was to speak English. I speak "psychiatristese" and everybody expects me to do it. Many of the psychiatrists I know who are interested in the city and are working with people concerned with urban problems also speak "psychiatristese." And nobody else understands what they are talking about. Certainly the mayors do not.

Mayors are hard to talk to. As I learned when I was with the Peace Corps, when you meet with Sargent Shriver you have to talk to him in five seconds. A mayor is the same way. I think we have a lot to learn in this area.

Right now the cities are in a crisis of fantastic dimensions. The Department of Housing and Urban Development is talking about giving the cities about $400 million for Model Cities Programs, and yet the city of New York alone wants a billion and a half the first year. And they need it and can use it. But our cities are "broke" in other ways too. They do not know how to pull their pieces and parts together.

In one city recently I saw a computer data system, about which I first talked to the mayor's assistant nine years ago. The idea then was to set up a data system which could tell you what was going on in the city at any time. The mayor's office discovered that there were about 60 or 70 data systems already in existence, all using their own information and definitions. No one had thought of pulling them together until then.

One fact psychiatrists have learned is that in times of social crisis people are susceptible to help. We also know it is at such moments that they are willing to change. If we can reach the mayors and the people concerned about the cities in their crises with assistance in the acute problems they are facing, they will begin to use us and we can help bring about change. I suggest that we begin to take them on as clients. We cannot wait for them to request our services, because they are not going to ask us. We must begin right now to fill in and be of assistance to them with the issues they are facing.

There is another crisis at present, which has happened in the last five months. A polarization is developing in our society. You can see it in California and in the East, with black militancy on one side and reaction on the other. This polarization is developing with such strong intensity that the communications between the two sides are disintegrating rapidly. When I started working with the Commission on Civil Disorders, we could not get the black militants to talk to the Commission. They did not want to talk. We had to see them secretly in back rooms. They said if anybody in their own group found out they were talking to us, they would be "finished."

Thus the critical problem is to maintain communications, to keep the avenues of communication open; because as the loss of communication and polarization grows, the possibility of solution diminishes. We all know this principle works also in terms of family welfare: the minute communication stops, the family unity begins to deteriorate. I am concerned because the temptation seems everywhere to be to find out ways of increasing the polarization. The popular demands about handling the riots today primarily concern the question of how to control the behavior of protesting people. And this sentiment increases the polarization.

I am asking psychiatrists to serve in a very unique capacity: that of bringing a little sense into this world of urban communication.

I want to close with some comparisons based on a trip I took to Israel right after the war in the summer of 1967. The most striking observation I made during my three weeks in Jerusalem was that the city had the same kind of problems that I see in every city in the United States—all the problems of urban organization, as well as a "race problem," in this case between the Oriental Jews, who make up about 70 per cent of the population and who have come from Africa and Asia, and the European, or Western, Jews.

Jerusalem has a very interesting choice ahead of it now. If the present polarization continues, the Oriental Jews may take over. They may very well replace the new Israel with the traditions and government of middle eastern countries. If on the other hand the European Jews begin to teach the Oriental Jews, if they begin to take them into our Western culture and give them Western skills, this 70 per cent may learn these skills so well that they still end up running the country, but by Western rules and as a Western nation.

The point I am trying to make about the world as it exists now is that the new militancy is presently the only choice open to our alienated. The present polarization presents only two sets of rules, with the other set being police control and concurrent apathy. Therefore, if our modern society is going to survive in its complexity, we have to come toward a new set of rules, which is equitable for all segments of our population.

There are going to have to be some radical changes before these new rules can emerge. The people from the world of the alienated have to learn. And like the Israeli I'd rather have them learn those rules and change our rules in the process than play the game by the rule of the jungle and the rule of polarization, which can only lead to utterly irreconcilable values.

Psychiatry can help to effect these changes by assisting the alienated people in learning our rules and our society as a whole in changing those rules which discriminate against this population. As "Distress in the City" verifies, the lack of communication between the impoverished and the city programs designed to assist them is ultimately responsible for many of the emotional disturbances—and their lack of treatment—which prevent these people from being an integral part of our urban society. The report is evidence of the need for psychiatry to change before we can hope for the plight of our urban poor to improve; it should be interpreted as a plea to psychiatry to take a greater part of the action in our cities.

LET'S TRY PREVENTION

꿈

LOYD W. ROWLAND [1]

The Louisiana Association for Mental Health

If, as Dr. Ryan's study shows, we are really not reaching emotionally disturbed persons at all with our present therapeutic program—and unless we are able to come up with some drastic additions to mental health personnel, which is unlikely—we had better get busy with new techniques. Let's try prevention! We have never done it, you know, at least not in a truly comprehensive way. And that is the approach which prevention must follow if we are to get results. Our efforts have always been spotty in terms of time and coverage. We have not tried any program of prevention for two generations or reached all the persons in any given category of our society. The expense will be far less if we try prevention and the results turn out to be much more to our liking. Anyway, we're not meeting the need with our present system, and one of the criteria of intelligence has always been the ability to vary one's problem-solving efforts.

Psychiatry is a precious commodity and should be concerned primarily with those persons who are mentally ill. Whatever

[1] Director of Education and Research.

psychiatrists have to say about prevention of emotional disturbance will be most welcome. But they have not evolved very much by way of methods that look toward the prevention of trouble. They know this and are becoming increasingly thoughtful about what can be done to prevent emotional disturbances.

Even if we continue along the same lines we have followed in the past, we will have to extend our efforts so as to include the skills of persons other than psychiatrists.

As Dr. Ryan's study indicates, clergymen represent a good resource, and they have been working at the matter of counseling for many generations. With not a great amount of psychological-psychiatric training they can be of even more use. It was once feared that the moralizing approach associated with ministers would inhibit the effectiveness of counseling by members of that profession, but such does not seem to be the case. They are increasingly useful. With the clergyman's theological role greatly beclouded these days, he can bring fresh enthusiasm to the "here and now" of emotional problems within his circle of influence.

If the theological personnel of the country are caring for so many emotionally disturbed people, it is perfectly obvious that in the training centers for them there must be far better training in personality development and counseling techniques than has been the case in the past. Many clergymen have had only a superficial smattering of psychology, and the sort they do have is of such an academic character as to be not very useful to them when they come to work with problem people. Thus the typical curriculum of the theological school, which includes Hebrew and Greek, systematic theology, homiletics, and church history, will have to have a great supplementation by way of training in the understanding of emotionally disturbed persons. Most clergymen can become skilled in the recognition of this area of need and can be a therapeutic source.

Mental health principles can become more deeply ingrained into the thinking of more professional people than we suppose.

Let me give an example to show how much psychiatric wisdom or insight—or whatever one may wish to call it—resides in visiting teachers and no doubt can be infused into many groups.

Some time ago, when I was in Europe, I was given French and Dutch pamphlets on parent education. I was particularly pleased with the illustrations in them, many of which were highly imaginative, rather abstract in nature, and showed children in problem situations of all kinds. There were enough cues in each sketch to suggest to discerning people the cause of the trouble. I couldn't read French and Dutch very well, but I was so attracted by the illustrations that I put them on slides and used a few of them one afternoon in what turned out to be a very interesting experiment.[2]

The visiting teachers of New Orleans had asked me to suggest some kind of program for one of their meetings. We worked out a plan to show slides and ask for interpretations. As it happened, the meeting was a fairly large one, with at least 60 to 70 visiting teachers. At the side of the room we seated a panel of experts—a psychiatrist, a school psychologist, a social worker, and a pediatrician.

What made our program unique was the time at which we allowed the panel to function. Our procedure was this: we would flash one of the sketches on the screen for about one-half minute, asking everyone in the audience to look at it and make his own interpretation of what the situation involved. Then we allowed *the audience first*, and *not the experts*, to interpret the illustrations. Participation began instantly, and it was difficult to provide time for everyone to express his opinion. Some very insightful interpretations were given. When the audience had no more opinions to express, we turned to the panel of experts for their interpretations.

[2] A more detailed account of this experiment may be found in *Ideas: Newsletter of the Committee for Mental Health Education*, ed. Joanna Nelle (Lincoln, Nebraska: Nebraska Psychiatric Institute), 1, no. 2 (1967): 3–4.

This was an interesting "twist," because usually the experts get the first chance at interpretation. The experts in this case really had nothing to add—at least, nothing very different—because the audience had already interpreted the sketches, and the panel looked a little helpless. What a reversal of procedure! Usually the experts exhaust the subject and then ask the audience if there are any questions, and often there are none. The silence makes the audience seem dull, but the real reason for it is simply that the speakers have covered all aspects of the subject.

It was a most interesting experience for the visiting teachers, because they seemed to develop very quickly the feeling that they were not without some insight themselves when it came to understanding human behavior. What they did not seem to realize was that, as the hour progressed, their interpretations began to be made more and more from what we might call the "mental health point of view." I think this change was due largely to the presence of the panel, which kept supplementing the mental health ideas or at least confirming those of the visiting teachers.

It is very gratifying to find the insights of a panel of professional persons anticipated by a lay group—at least, what is called "a lay group"; such an occurrence indicates the extent to which we have been effective in teaching mental health principles and suggests that we might be even more effective if we could get our ideas around more generally. Now, I know the critic will say: "But this was the compilation of the wisdom of all the people in the audience." Well, that's true and it doesn't mean that any one individual in the group would necessarily have come forth with as good an answer as the group was able to supply. On the other hand, there are doubtless many good ideas that were never expressed.

Well-known recent studies made in Washington, D. C., have indicated that housewives can be trained as counselors and that they do an excellent job. This finding doubtless means that a great deal of counseling wisdom was already in the minds of the trainees. They had not learned everything "from scratch." I have known many housewives, as you probably have, whose understandings of emotional problems and social situations were quite equal to that of the average psychiatrist or any other professional who purports to understand human beings.

Even with the training of supplementary personnel, however, it appears that we shall never be able to help all those who have emotional problems—those in the upper quartile who have manifest emotional disturbances.

But what about the next quartile? This group undoubtedly has within it people who are just below the limen of demonstrable difficulty. They are the ones who repress their children, make the life of a spouse intolerable, barely keep a job, and feel they always have to be "different" just for the sake of being so.

If with our present methods we can't help the upper quartile of persons having emotional difficulties, we can't do much for the second group; and the only method that seems to remain open to us is to build into our culture the elements of prevention.

But this approach requires that we know the causes of disturbance and that some sort of reasonable solutions have been found.

The fact is that we don't have any very "hard-nosed" research to support our contention that emotional disturbance is preventable. However, the term "hard-nosed" is one that has professional overtones, and its meaning is relative, in a way that reminds me of the concluding pages of T. V. Smith's autobiography, *A Non-Existent Man*,[3] in which he lists the seven observations he has made with regard to men and society. The first of these is "No man is an S.O.B. to himself." The corollary to that would be that every investigator is "hard-nosed" unto himself, and it is much easier to be "hard-nosed" in some disciplines than in others. Those who have a clear mandate to use a mathematical-experimental ap-

[3] T. V. Smith, *A Non-Existent Man* (Austin, Texas: The University of Texas Press, 1962), p. 251.

proach, such as physicists, look down their noses—and I don't mean to mix metaphors—at the biologists, whose experimental approach is not as rigid as that of the physicists. The biologists have a measure of distrust in the "scientific standards" of the psychologists, who in their turn are amused at the sociologists, who say the anthropologists have the "softest noses" of all.

As a matter of fact, many programs have been initiated without any very complete "hard-nosed" conclusions, regardless of the area being considered. Physicians have to live every day with the problem of being unsure. The need to act without complete certainty extends even to the changing of the institutions of our society.

In the United States the orphans' home is disappearing as an institution. I live within half a mile of three orphans' homes that have been closed within the last twenty years. Now, why did these orphans' homes close? Perhaps the answer is that about a generation ago investigators began to discover that children deteriorated *intellectually* in the absence of the kind of stimulation which is present in homes. They found that IQ goes down in proportion to length of stay in an orphans' home. And this was discovered at the time when the IQ was "king." (Professionals now tend to downgrade the importance of IQ, but they keep using it and depend upon it as a useful index.) When these studies were widely talked about, it was not long until orphans' homes began to be closed—first the weak ones and then the stronger ones. Finally, those that remained were mostly the endowed ones, and these are hard to change in any case.

It was found that children do better in adoptive homes and that plenty of such homes are available.

Now, the point is that the investigators did not have complete information, but they proceeded along what seemed to be better approaches, and apparently they were right.

Here is another example. For a good many years now, studies have been indicating that a very young child who has been cared for only by his mother, with no "mother-substitutes," is greatly disturbed if he loses his mother or if she is gone from his presence during the better part of his waking hours.

This finding was summarized very well by Dr. John Bowlby in his book on maternal care and the mental health of children, published in 1951.[4] I talked with him in the summer of 1956 and, to quote him approximately, he said, "There's something about the second half of the first year which makes it very important for the mother to be with her child." Others say that if the youngster is handled by *several people* from infancy, it does not make too much difference when the mother is absent. However, we must face the realistic fact that in our western culture, which features mobility and nuclear families, there usually aren't a lot of people to feed and clothe a baby and look after him, so that normally a mother *is* missed greatly if she is not fairly constantly available.

As a result of Dr. Bowlby's monograph, which was written under the aegis of the World Health Organization, better institutions for babies throughout the land developed practices whereby each baby was given individual attention several times during the day and different persons looked after him, not just one person who might discontinue doing so. Individual attention means more than going by the crib and speaking to each child. It means picking him up, cuddling him, carrying him around, and showing love for him and real interest. This process is in striking contrast to the so-called sanitary procedure once followed, whereby children were fed, changed, put back on the bed, and allowed to look at the ceiling—instead of being talked to, fussed over, petted, and encouraged to babble and respond in other ways.

Now, the studies on which this change in ways of handling children is based may not be sufficiently "hard-nosed" to suit some investigators, but the new practice has spread and is more

[4] John Bowlby, *Maternal Care and Mental Health* (Geneva: World Health Organization, 1951).

satisfying to caretakers, who are now convinced of its effectiveness.

In proceeding with the development of an educational program, we have to go ahead with our best insights, without always having complete "hard-nosed" support of our hopes. Certainly we don't always have an *experimental* base from which to begin. We do what we do because it seems "self-evident," or we simply proceed on the basis of what we think will help. There were no complete data, so far as I know, to support the Head Start program, but there are children who do not know "middle-class" English—which is and must be the language of the schools. Such children do not know the school pronunciation of common words. When they talk, it is difficult for the teacher to understand. They have not used chalk or a blackboard—or sometimes even knives and forks. Many have been beaten and pushed around by their parents and older siblings until they are hesitant to show any initiative in problem solving.

Attempts are being made to evaluate, guide, and improve the Head Start program, but nobody now seems to question the good it does deprived children.

Without laboring the point too much, here is another illustration. The value of kindergarten is very difficult to demonstrate. Children who have been to kindergarten do not learn reading and arithmetic more readily than children who have not attended kindergarten. Yet the growth of the kindergarten movement continues, and both parents and teachers concede its worth. Parents feel that the time has come for a child to have wider social experience when he is five years of age and that many emotional blockings to learning will be avoided if he can be with children in a play situation for a year before he settles down to learning the curriculum for elementary education that the school has set up for him.

We sometimes use this incomplete kind of "self-evidence" in initiating mental health programs. For example, no accurate statistical study is needed to see that men in retirement are restive these days. Just talk to a few of them. Or better still, talk to their wives. A sample will be convincing.

I. What Are the Approaches We Would Use in a Preventive Program?

Manipulating the environment is essential in any preventive program. For example, there has been some extremely interesting work done on crowding in animals. The work was initiated with rats and has been extended into higher orders of mammals with the same results: it is possible to get too many individuals in the same area for good emotional health, even though their basic needs are met. The time may well come when it will be possible to work out by means of a formula the maximal number of persons who may live within a given area. This formula will be modified, of course, by the number of floors in an apartment building and the number of compensating open spaces in those apartment buildings at all levels. For example, if there were a play room in the center of each floor in a large apartment building, the space on which the building sits would be greatly "expanded." The time may also come when people will be forbidden to crowd into spaces which are inadequate in terms of square footage. Crowding may well be partly responsible for our riots in the 1960's, though most investigators would emphasize that it is only *part* of the problem.

We know that poverty creates emotional disturbances. In this case, elemental needs are not met. Poverty makes for conflicts between members of the family with respect to how and what expenditures shall be made. Living close to or below the fiscal limen is too hard for many families. They begin to produce disturbed individuals.

Immediately we pose the question of whether any of the emotional disturbance in the 20–25 per cent of the population of which Dr. Ryan speaks might have been prevented. This is a fair question to ask, especially when it is clear that present mental health services are *not* reaching those persons who are emotionally disturbed. One wants to know whether large-scale efforts could be made which would result in an educational process that in turn would give us less emotional disturbance. The energy we have put into training for the handling of emotionally disturbed people has never been put into prevention. We wait until the individual "snaps," as we say, and then we try to restore him. Surely, by all the observations we have been able to make with regard to people and things, it is better to prevent than to try to cure.

Our society must move ahead and seek aggressively the conditions that promote mental health and that avoid emotional disturbance. To consider a parallel situation, I have talked with a number of people who have been in forestry work, and they report that one of the causes of forest fires is complete boredom on the part of people who live in the area. The forest fire affords excitement. Knowing these reports, it is the better part of wisdom to provide entertainment and excitement other than that which forest fires can give. While this situation is only an analogy, it seems to me to be a very close one and to have a solution which is applicable in principle to mental health problems in our cities.

Our purpose is to saturate the whole population with foreknowledge of some of the problems they are to face and to supply them with partial solutions. With such guidance life may be much richer, happier, and more rewarding.

Assuming we wish to try out a plan for anticipating emotional difficulties and preventing them, what are some guideposts we should follow in developing methods of helpfulness?

Here are some suggestions:

1. We should try to reach *all people*. This calls for far larger programs than have ever been envisioned before. However, there are precedents. In our society we think it important that every-

body be able to read and write, and we will even coerce a juvenile if need be—we have compulsory school attendance laws.

In much the same way, we should try to think in terms of improving the mental health of everyone. But such a goal does not mean there is a single approach to improving the mental health of all persons in the population. Instead, the most efficient way seems to be to try to approach people in the area of their present need or their expected need. We call this "working with homogeneous, highly motivated groups." We reach as many people as we can who have the same need and have it strongly. For example, all parents have about the same problems when they have their first child, whether they live in the ghetto or on the avenue. College students have much the same problems of adjustment, whether they work in the cafeteria or drive an expensive, imported sport car.

High school students have much the same problems of learning to make good choices, of learning to live with their bodies, of "breaking away" from their parents, of becoming responsible adults. These students should be taught the realities of marriage: that it's not always blissful, as some romantic literature depicts, but that babies come and they cry in the middle of the night and must be cared for; that dishes are an unending chore; that everyone has to "clean up his own mess" if the household is to proceed with any smoothness at all; that there may be conflicts, tears, unfairness, unwillingness to share, harsh words. Can they survive this? Knowledge beforehand would help. It is a great experience for senior high school students to sit down at a long table and talk over these problems as a group, having read something about them beforehand.

For the adolescent there is still status in the mail box. He doesn't get as much mail as adults do. His name has not been placed on dozens of mailing lists throughout the country. He even treasures his "junk mail" and is resentful when somebody opens it. If he receives first-class letters, he treasures them very much, and we can depend upon it that he will read and consider what comes to him in such a fashion. By thus using the mail we might cover an entire population of high school students at any grade level.

Another group that is reachable and in need of anticipatory guidance is the college senior—and he too is available: we can get his name and address. We are saying more and more these days that a college education is essential to real success. We are giving young people a rather grandiose notion of what will follow college. Instead, we should be a great deal more realistic about what actually happens after graduation.

As an example, many college students find that recruiters come to the campuses and are keen to interview them and get them employed by their companies. Let's say the field is engineering, some special branch of it—perhaps aeronautical engineering. What the students do not realize is that the companies employ many persons with the full intent of weeding out some of these graduates a couple of years later, thus leaving them without employment. The second-string companies then take them on and they get a drop in self-esteem and perhaps even in salary. College students should be prepared for this. It takes place in all kinds of businesses and industries.

Young people ought to know of these competitions in our society. They should also know there is a great deal of detail work that must be done in every position. Quite a few years ago I was about to be offered a position as Examiner for the Chicago Public Schools. I went to the late Professor L. L. Thurstone and asked him about the position, saying, "I am afraid this work would become very monotonous." His answer was quick. He said, "It would be up to you to see that it did not become so. Any job can become monotonous." We ought to teach young people that much of the work they do for a living will have a great sameness. There are not, as the undergraduate is led to believe, many jobs which provide opportunity for originality; and very few jobs permit the average college graduate to dream up schemes and plans, as he is led in his undergraduate days to believe he will be able to.

When we teach college students such facts about employment, we are not making "a bunch of wise guys" out of them. Instead, we are forewarning them of the nature of present-day employment.

2. In a program of prevention we should use whatever techniques are appropriate. Naturally, these days we all think of television and its enormous popularity. But can we depend upon it as a source of mental health teaching? We can't, except indirectly. The programming is now determined largely by the networks, which are concerned chiefly with the number of viewers and very little with their education. Perhaps more of the programs could be slanted in the direction of mental health needs. The program "Father Knows Best," which ran for many years, was a beautiful depiction of family life, and many viewers must have learned something about handling their problems from seeing the situations presented. The present program "My Three Sons" is a fine example of a family doing its best, making good adjustments under difficult conditions.

However, until such a time as we have a national television network with teaching programs that go beyond entertainment per se, we can not expect much from this resource. We await with interest the use of closed-circuit television for teaching large numbers of people.

Consider radio. All one has to do if he wants to know why radio is not used more for teaching purposes is to tune in all the stations he can, from one end of the dial to the other. He will quickly turn off the set. Radio still has educational status in some countries, but not in the United States. There are a few good programs, but they are hard to find.

We might continue with this consideration of the "mass media," but I think they are of little use to us, in their present form of programming, for mental health teaching. For one thing, we don't know who watches or listens to them, and it is easy to overstate the case for a medium that supposedly reaches so many people.

3. The printing press still has status with most people. We tend to think that once something is printed it is "the law and the gospel"—i.e., that it must be correct. Just why this is the case, we do not know, but we don't as a rule challenge something that is printed. Even a writer gets a bit of this feeling. He may be ever so dissatisfied with his material while it is in manuscript form, but once it is printed, it looks "pretty good." Also, we can control printed matter. We know to whom it goes and in what quantity. Knowing in advance to whom the material is going enables us to know how to prepare it and lends some certainty that it will be read and studied.

The impact of printed material may be very great, depending upon the individual's need at the moment and the status fashion in which it is introduced to him.

4. Another thing we should do, having thought out a program and put it into operation, is to continue it a long, long time. Nothing is more disconcerting than the fly-by-night pattern of the mental health education programs we adopt. We find a play that is good for parents of second-grade pupils. We give it one time and then stop, thinking we have performed a good service. We have, but why not give it to all the parents who have children in the second grade in your city; why not give it again the next year and the next, for at least ten years? We don't use in a systematic way the materials we have in mental health. Just because a film gets old, for example, we tend not to use it. But every parent should see the film *Preface to a Life* a few times. I never tire of seeing it. Every person who is about to be discharged from a mental hospital should see *Bitter Welcome* once or twice. Any given mental hospital should have the routine

practice of showing this film to all persons who are getting ready to go home. We have many fine teaching materials if we would only use them.

Two years ago I saw Elizabeth Carmichael of the University of Alabama hold a hundred sixth-grade boys spellbound for an hour as she demonstrated models showing the growth and birth of a baby, and the response of the boys was so intelligent! Undoubtedly many anxieties on reproduction were lessened, and the boys all seemed to leave with an aura of good feeling about the birth process.

My first questions after seeing this demonstration were: "How many other boys and girls in your state will see this? What are your plans for showing this from year to year to *all* youngsters who reach the sixth-grade level?"

To summarize, we must use whatever devices are appropriate in mental health education. Sometimes this means discussion groups, films, printed material, talks, closed-circuit television— whatever the genius of the age comes up with, just so it reaches as many persons as possible in the group to which an appeal is being made.

When all these efforts have been added together, we will have reached the goal of our endeavors. It will not be reached, however, by a single approach but by various means with special groups.

II. Evaluation

The professional community has the responsibility of asking whether a program is effective, but it does not have the right to do so with a preconceived methodology for measuring this effectiveness.

It is my purpose here to set down some ways, formal and informal, of demonstrating the effectiveness of the programs we have been working with in the Louisiana Association for Mental Health during recent years. Let us start off with an example of police education.[5]

Some years ago a friend of mine asked me to help with the apprehension of a mentally ill young woman who was causing disturbance in his church. There was a psychiatrist in the church who observed her, and without her knowledge commitment papers were prepared; it remained only for her to be identified and apprehended by the police and taken to the hospital. She had no family to assist with handling her case, which was a fairly serious one.

By prearrangement my friend and I and two young police officers approached her as she was about to enter her house. She was asked to sit on the porch in a swing, which she did. Now, the purpose of this story is to report the behavior of the young officers for the few minutes that followed.

They removed their caps and told the young woman they had a writ from the coroner's office to take her to a hospital. They attempted to persuade her to go with them in the squad car, but she refused. One officer sat on a banister of the porch and the other, in his eagerness to clarify the facts, squatted down into a sort of sitting position and explained every detail, but she still refused to go to the hospital.

The officers gave her the ultimatum that either she could go with them "like a lady" in the squad car or they would send for the wagon. Finally they did call the wagon and both the squad car and the wagon were drawn up in front of the house. Still she refused to go, so they politely, but firmly, took hold of her arms and led her down the porch steps, offering her the alternative still of going in the squad car or the wagon. She started in the

[5] This account is given with the permission of the *FBI Law Enforcement Bulletin*, where a somewhat fuller report appeared. (See Loyd W. Rowland, "Care is Necessary in Apprehending the Mentally Ill," *FBI Law Enforcement Bulletin* 30, no. 1 [January 1961]: 3–5.)

direction of the squad car and then began to resist. They opened the door of the wagon and deftly slipped her inside, after quickly examining her purse for any dangerous objects which she might carry along.

When it was all over, I asked one of the young officers where they had learned about mental illness and the handling of mentally ill people. He replied, "Oh, we have a little manual over in the department, called 'How to Recognize and Handle Abnormal People.' " This was a great experience for me, for I was the person who had had the idea of preparing this manual and was coauthor of it.

Another instance of the effect of mental health teaching on police was reported to us by Irene Wilson Laune, the editor of the film *The Mask*. She wanted to get some feeling for police operations, and therefore asked a sheriff of a small town not far from New York City if she could come and make observations. Her plan was to "stick around" and see how things went. The sheriff said, "You know, my wife is a psychiatric nurse and works here in the department. Time was when the officers would come with a disturbed patient and would say to her in a loud voice, 'Here, take this nut off my hands!' But no more. Now they slip up to her and say quietly, 'I think this man is in bad shape. See what you can do for him.' So you can see that our teaching these men and showing them films has done some good."

Until such time as more sophisticated studies are made of police education, anecdotal instances of this sort will have to suffice. Meanwhile, we are confident of the good results that come from police education in mental health practices.

Confirmation of the effectiveness of an educational program often comes from most unexpected sources and sometimes in most unusual ways. For example, the City of Berlin is using our American program called *Pierre the Pelican*. Two years ago the program had been in use for a total of six years, so that the first children whose parents had received this material were entering school. The *Berliner Zeitung*, one of the large papers of Berlin, ran an article in which attention was called to letters it was receiving from parents who complained that their children were being roughly handled at the time physical examinations were being given as they entered school. Dr. Ruth Mattheis, who is associated with the Ministry of Health of the City of Berlin and was formerly a school physician, was incensed when this story appeared in the paper. She called up the editor to inquire, "How many of these letters have been received—one or two?" The answer was, "We have received 150 of them." This was a great surprise, as nothing like it had ever happened before and there was no other factor that could account for these complaints, which came from *all twelve districts* of the City and apparently without any collaboration whatsoever. The only explanation was that a different level of expectation—different values, as we say —had been built into the parents by the *Pierre the Pelican* series. A study of the records showed that almost exactly one-half of the children entering the first grade had parents who had received the *Pierre the Pelican* series, yet almost all (95 per cent) of the *complaints had come from this group. In other words, the "Pierre" parents complained nineteen times as often as the parents who had not received the series.*

The effects of teaching on an entire culture can be seen, especially when that culture is somewhat different from the one in which we grew up. Here is a good instance.

My wife and I have a son who is a linguist and, while in the process of acquiring the use of various languages, he learned Arabic. In order to do this he went to the old city of Aleppo in Syria and found a young man there who would share his apartment and teach him Arabic. In this old city very little English is used and this was a good place to learn to speak the language. Our son made an incidental remark, when he was discussing the life and customs of the people, that "Probably there is not a pig in all Syria."

I went through the Koran and found four references to "swine meat" as being forbidden food. Here, of course, we have an institution, the religion of Islam, back of the printed word, sustaining the use of the Koran.

It is surprising how long some of the practices that were initiated by religious groups exist and how strong they are. When a Jewish home for elderly persons was recently established in New Orleans, acknowledgement of the religion was made in the plan: a double kitchen was built into the installation, so that meat and milk would not be cooked in the same utensils. This was done to accord with centuries-old teachings of the Jewish faith.

Similarly, in Christian churches the prominence given to the Bible is evident to all who attend them.

If one has further doubts about the influence of the printed word, let him look at the television and note the fanatical youth of China holding their red books in the air—the books which are described as "the thought of Mao Tse-tung."

All these examples represent the effects of teaching a book— but by an institution. If we ever evolve a "book" of mental health teachings and an institution to support its use, we will be in a situation not unlike political and religious groups. In the case of mental health it might be better to have the book without the supporting institution!

Sometimes, although we always try, we can not demonstrate the worth of a program statistically; but all we have to do to discover its value is to ask the recipients for their opinions of it. The effectiveness of this procedure is nowhere more dramatically reflected than in a study made by Greenberg and others of the early *Pierre the Pelican* program, in which changes in feeding practices could not be detected as a result of parents reading the series.[6] But when 2496 cards were mailed to a sample of parents of

[6] See B. G. Greenberg *et al.*, "A Method of Evaluating the Effectiveness of Health Education Literature," *The American Journal of Public Health* 43 (September 1953): 1147-61.

83 counties in North Carolina, 50.7 per cent of the total number was returned and "every answer was in favor of continuing the series." (This is the largest percentage of returns for free literature we have ever heard of.) Furthermore, the authors continue, "Of those returning the cards, about 90 per cent answered that they were saving the pamphlets, and, without being asked, 82 per cent volunteered that they had found the *Pierre* pamphlets helpful." Later I asked Professor Greenberg for his cards and scaled these opinions by the method of equal-appearing intervals. The statement "I find these pamphlets very helpful" was the most representative one. It is hard to deny the validating quality of such remarks by the recipients.

I am sorry that through the years we have not kept all the letters which have been sent to us by parents, expressing their satisfaction at receiving the *Pierre the Pelican* series. We have kept many hundreds of them, and a physician staff member at the State Department of Health answers them, with particular regard for those letters which present problems and want help. We have made up books of the most interesting of them to send to the sponsors of the program. In Berlin the Arbeitskreis Neue Erziehung has lined the walls of its hallways with photographs of their children sent by young parents in appreciation of *"Peter Pelikan,"* as the service is called there.

Another criterion of worth is what the authorities say. A wise parent can not always explain fully why he wishes a child to perform in a certain way, though he can always try. In much the same way, the authority in the field of mental health education, presumed to know more than the layman, cannot always say what services he thinks will help. If pushed for explanation, he can give his opinion of the worth of the services and his reason for that opinion. Even if he gives an incomplete reason, it is likely to have some validity.

We think the best really "hard-nosed" study that has been made of the old *Pierre the Pelican* educational program (when it comprised only twelve pamphlets) was done by twenty graduate students in social work at Tulane University as a thesis project.[7] The following conclusions were submitted.

> When the *Pierre the Pelican* pamphlets are distributed routinely to parents of firstborn children they are read widely by both mother and father. There is clear evidence that the *Pierre the Pelican* series is an effective device in mass education along the lines of prevention in mental health. A series of questions asked of parents who had received the literature, as over against the same questions asked of those who had not, shows that the members of the former group are more likely to accept principles of child care commonly advocated by experts in the field. Even where the results are small enough to be inconclusive, they are "in the direction of" favoring the parents who have been sent the series.

A research report made in Michigan in general confirmed the results of this study,[8] but that made by Greenberg did not find positive results.

In mental health education it is only fair to ask for a reasonable amount of time to pass before we are required to assess what we have done. Biologists are permitted to study many generations of plant and animal life before conclusions are reached. Many biological experiments are even carried from one generation of scientists to the next. Psychologists consider important the so-called longitudinal studies, where individuals are studied from birth until maturity and beyond. Mental health educators should be given the same long-term opportunity to study the effects of any given mental health practices.

[7] See Loyd W. Rowland, "A First Evaluation of the *Pierre the Pelican* Mental Health Pamphlets," *The Louisiana Mental Health Studies* 1, no. 1 (November 1948): 1–22.

[8] Edward A. Bilitzke *et al.*, "A Report of Some Aspects of the Effectiveness of the *Pierre the Pelican* Mental Health Pamphlets" (Lansing: Michigan State Department of Mental Health, November 1952). Mimeographed.

We must be careful that our efforts in mental health education do not conflict with larger social and political values. For a long time now we have been encouraging *individual growth in decision making*. But, in the United States at least, this is something that must take into consideration the functioning of representative democracy. The clash appears when we have on the one hand elected officials who are governing the country and on the other hand "individuals" who choose to try to force their opinions by bizarre behavior, parades, clashes with the police, and riots. We have to assess what we are teaching to see at what point too much freedom for individual decision making impinges on the rights of others.

We even run the risk of survival into a future culture of slogans or ways of reacting which we have taught and which will not be acceptable to future society. A good example is the adage "Spare the rod and spoil the child," which was probably highly acceptable centuries ago. At the present time almost everyone approves the idea of discipline in childhood—and adulthood—but we look with concern at the parent who punishes his child too much by whipping, and many of the states have recently—and without opposition—passed legislation to protect children from being battered.

We hopefully assume that with an increase of knowledge there will be increasing insight into what it takes to make a mentally healthy person and that this insight will be followed by appropriate behavior.

Always it must be kept in mind that the general goal toward which we are striving is to *prevent* those situations which distort the individual and make him ineffective.

And so we do the best we know and can.

REFERENCES

Bilitzke, Edward A., *et al.* "A Report of Some Aspects of the Effectiveness of the *Pierre the Pelican* Mental Health Pamphlets."

Mimeographed. Lansing, Michigan: Michigan State Department of Mental Health, November 1952.

Bowlby, John. *Maternal Care and Mental Health*. Geneva: World Health Organization, 1951.

Greenberg, B. G.; Harris, Mary Ellen; MacKinnon, C. Francis; and Chipman, Sidney S. "A Method of Evaluating the Effectiveness of Health Education Literature." *The American Journal of Public Health* 43 (1953): 1147–61.

Nelle, Joanna, ed. *Ideas: Newsletter of the Committee for Mental Health Education* (Lincoln, Nebraska: Nebraska Psychiatric Institute) 1, no. 2 (1967).

Rowland, Loyd W. "Care is Necessary in Apprehending the Mentally Ill." *FBI Law Enforcement Bulletin* 30, no. 1 (1961): 3–5.

Rowland, Loyd W. "A First Evaluation of the *Pierre the Pelican* Mental Health Pamphlets." *The Louisiana Mental Health Studies* 1 (1948): 1–22.

Smith, T. V. *A Non-Existent Man*. Austin, Texas: University of Texas Press, 1962.

THE BOSTON MENTAL HEALTH SURVEY: A CONTEXT FOR INTERPRETATION

❀

FRANKLYN N. ARNHOFF [1]

National Institute of Mental Health [2]

The sobering and impressive results of Dr. Ryan's work document the parallel between the broader national health scene, as discussed in the *Report of the National Advisory Commission on Health Manpower* (1967), and the area referred to as "mental health." General health services to the poor, the aged, and the Negro continue to be inadequate or nonexistent and grow worse rather than better. In the mental health area, long after the pioneering work of Hollingshead and Redlich,[3] those viewed as mentally disturbed, both in hospital and out, are still receiving differential attention as a function of their social and economic status, chronological age, and/or racial characteristics. Viewed in its broadest context, the Boston Mental Health Survey adds another systematic account of current welfare service and its deficiencies. After years of legislation, studies, surveys, and polemics, plus the expenditure of countless billions of dollars, there are still

[1] Chief, Manpower and Analytic Studies Branch.

[2] The opinions expressed are those of the individual author and do not necessarily reflect the position or policies of the NIMH.

[3] See A. B. Hollingshead and F. C. Redlich, *Social Class and Mental Illness* (New York: John Wiley & Sons, Inc., 1958).

millions of persons in trouble with no place to go and no help available.

As far as mental health services are concerned, increase in the prevalence of psychosis, with a concomitant overtaxing of facilities, is not the reason for these deficiencies and cannot be offered as even partial explanation. There is still no evidence to contradict the Goldhammer and Marshall data, which indicate no change in rates of psychosis over the past century.[4] As Mencher has observed: "The increase in social services required for the modern urban community probably cannot be accounted for, except to a relatively modest degree, by an accelerated incidence of individual and social breakdown. The absence or rejection of primary group support systems and changing expectations of adequate care account for much of the increased demand." [5]

Since World War II and the explosive growth of the mental health field, a manpower shortage has been seen as a major limiting factor in service delivery, and this has been a point of continued iteration. The massive steps taken to develop educational and training programs have resulted in a continuous supply of trained professionals,[6] but there still exists not a constant gap but a *growing* gap between available supply and perceived need. The Boston metropolitan area has one of the highest ratios of mental health personnel and facilities to population in the country, and still it is seen as understaffed. As explanations for this

[4] See H. Goldhammer and A. Marshall, *Psychosis and Civilization* (Glencoe, Illinois: The Free Press, 1953).

[5] S. Mencher, "Social Trends, Social Policy and Manpower" (Paper given at the Institute on Research Approaches to Manpower Problems in Social Welfare Services to Children and Families, University of Minnesota, Duluth Campus, August 1964), mimeographed, p. 3.

[6] See F. N. Arnhoff, "Realities and Mental Health Manpower," *Mental Hygiene* 52 (1968): 181–89; and F. N. Arnhoff *et al.*, "The Mental Health Fields: An Overview of Growth and Development," in *Manpower for Mental Health*, ed. F. N. Arnhoff, E. A. Rubinstein, and J. C. Speisman (Chicago: Aldine Publishing Company, 1969).

worsening situation, two basic phenomena emerge. One, of course, is the growing population, which reached 200 million in 1967 and is expected to be at about 300 million in the year 2000—an increase of one-half again in the next 31 years. A second, more immediately relevant, is that the definition of mental health has continued to expand, with concomitant expansion of conceptions of need and demand. Thus, the goals for provision of services have not remained at a constant ratio commensurate with population growth and professional manpower production but rather have tended to increase disproportionately. A rather common phenomenon can be observed at work: the tendency for supply to create its own demand with the result that the more hospitals, clinics, and services provided, the more patients and clients there are to demand service.

These two general points serve as the orientation for my remarks about this survey. Since the study was conducted in 1961–62, a vast amount of legislation, activity, and mental health involvement has transpired in the areas loosely referred to as poverty, urban affairs, social welfare, health services delivery, and racial equality. The problems of poverty, in particular, have been focused upon by the mental health professions and are viewed as antecedents of mental illness. To a very great extent the Boston survey is a study of poverty and urban affairs and is quite current in that respect. My remarks, therefore, are addressed to a current context of interpretation prevalent in the mental health field, a context with which it can be assumed the current study will be found quite compatible. Since I find this context and orientation quite incompatible with broader perspectives and needs, some hopefully prophylactic caveats and considerations will be introduced.

To go back to the expanding conceptions and definition of "mental health," a brief historical note is in order. Recall that the mental hygiene movement was initially concerned with mental illness—the major psychoses. Over time, due to the frightening nature of mental illness and the stigma attached to such conditions, the term "mental health" came into vogue in discussions of mental illness. This term has been ever broadened to include an increasing range of phenomena and is often used as if synonymous with total human behavior. This has been due in part to increasing sophistication in our knowledge of, attitudes toward, and way of handling the psychological components of human social functioning and in part to our continued ignorance as to the etiology and developmental antecedents of psychosis and other major behavioral disturbances. Questions as to whether neurosis and psychosis are continuous or orthogonal, whether early disturbance leads to later increased severity, and so forth, remain as yet unanswered. However, as the spectrum of behaviors potentially relevant was broadened, concepts of prophylaxis and early diagnosis and treatment were introduced as meaningful analogues to traditional disease approaches.

Still, the environmental and social factors in the development of behavior tended to be neglected in America until the late 1940's and 1950's in preference for individual psychodynamics, adjustment, and self-improvement—factors more compatible with American culture and the dominant protestant ethic.[7] Concerns for prevention in any broad social sense were minimal, and efforts were directed primarily toward individual improvement and treatment. As social scientists and public health specialists became incorporated into the mental health movement, however, emphasis upon prevention increased, and environmental factors, particularly social factors, received growing attention. This change in focus was critically reflected in the final report of the Joint Commission on Mental Illness and Health (1961), which felt that

[7] See N. Sanford, "The Prevention of Mental Illness," in *Handbook of Clinical Psychology*, ed. B. B. Wolman (New York: McGraw-Hill, Inc., 1965), pp. 1378–1400.

the mental health movement was overemphasizing prevention at the expense of treatment of major mental illness—the major psychoses and chronic mental disease. [8]

Since attempts at univocal definition of the term "mental health" have been unfruitful to date, no attempt will be made here to restrict its meaning. I will use the term in its broadest connotation, that of human behavior, and will use the term "mental illness" when psychosis and the major disabling neuroses are what is meant. This distinction is particularly meaningful in view of current societal trends and movements as well as the conceptual developments within the mental health field itself. These trends are epitomized by Ryan:

> The direct relationship between social problems and mental health is not only becoming more and more clear; it is increasingly becoming a matter of concern to thoughtful persons in the field. The stressful effects of poverty, poor housing, unemployment, racial discrimination, and inadequate schools are evident in many instances of emotional disturbance. There is a great deal of sentiment in favor of mental health professionals and interested citizens taking a much more active role in dealing with these issues (p. 64).

This brief quote accents the necessity for distinguishing between human behavior in general and those conditions which have traditionally been viewed as requiring the intervention and assistance of mental health professionals. The distinction, of course, is crude and overlaps at the margins, but in the absence of the etiologic, developmental data alluded to previously it may permit a better perspective to assess and interpret this study, the current mental health efforts, and future directions of effort.

While more will be said on this point later, it is sufficient to say here that the definition and use of these terms or labels are not

[8] Joint Commission on Mental Illness and Health, *Action for Mental Health* (New York: Basic Books, Inc., 1961).

merely an academic exercise; the definition of mental health and/or illness and assumptions as to etiology and course determine the scope of the problem, the differential roles and responsibilities of the "mental health" professions vis-a-vis other groups and society in general, the manpower specifications and requirements to deal with the problems, and last, but by no means least, the underlying social philosophy guiding these efforts.

The preceding discussion relates to the Boston Mental Health Survey in a very direct and critical fashion. It is apparent from the results that considerably more than mental health services, no matter how defined, are at issue. Although the study was designed, conducted, and reported under the aegis of mental health, it relates to, and is concerned with, the entire conception of social welfare and delivery of services to people in need. From the perspective of any system based upon severity of need for assistance, it is clear that not only have priorities often broken down, but in many instances they have never been developed.

As reported, the study criterion was "emotional disturbance," defined as being of "sufficient magnitude to interfere to an obvious degree with normal functioning" (p. 4). This definition is certainly imprecise, and the lack of specification does not allow for the formulation of problem-centered analysis. From the examples given, however, as well as from the discussion, it is evident that these problems run the gamut of human behavioral upheaval and that the aggregate term "emotionally disturbed" masks the etiologic basis and divergent nature of the difficulties which have been assessed and described on the basis of their affective expression. Thus, data on the expected divergence in social classes, life situational problems, economic and occupational status, and, most certainly, cognitive and intellectual differences are not available for scrutiny. So too, the five categories of persons for whom service is not generally available are not unidimensional and/or mutually exclusive but rather are groupings by age, socioeconomic status, and psychiatric status (roughly defined); the needed and specific services required would not necessarily be the same for all these categories of people. Racial factors are not specified, nor is the factor of length of residence in the area (necessary to assess into-city migration). Since the report given is in itself a summary and such data may be available for the study proper, I do not wish to appear overly critical but merely to state the roughness of these groupings, which necessarily precludes specific analyses.

While these are limiting factors for some purposes, the focus and mechanisms of the study are indicative of many current concerns and activities. My objection is to the "mental health" framework which guides and orients this and so many similar studies; it is frequently misleading and, I believe, actually inhibitory to maximal, corrective efforts. The latter point will be returned to and amplified in a succeeding section. On the positive side, the study was conducted under the auspices and coordination of three mental health groups, and, as reported, has led to greater coordination and enabling legislation for expanded mental health activities.

These accomplishments should not be demeaned or minimized, since coordination of such activities is sorely needed. Such accomplishments notwithstanding, the continued focus on health, particularly mental health, in endeavors which involve a complete range of human problems and behavior (and the limiting of the study to the emotional component of behavior at that) remains an inappropriate emphasis and approach.

The term "health" has little value for precise planning or for addressing definitive issues. Its utility in medicine serves for general communication and little else. For some years the medical profession and various related groups were quite concerned with concepts of health, particularly positive health, and considerable effort was expended in an attempt to arrive at meaningful definitions and criteria of good health. It was agreed rather early that more was involved than mere absence of demonstrable disease; but, from this point on, the issue bogged down and proved rather fruitless. This quest lost its appeal, and research on specific conditions and disease entities dealing with etiology and therapeutics has proved more rewarding.

Mental health has followed the same pattern to some extent, at least as far as the initial stage is concerned, except that the global term has even less consensus than does the term "physical health." The problems and behaviors involved under the term "mental health" cover an almost total range of human experience and function. Since human behavior involves ethical, moral, religious, and social values, to date it has been impossible to extricate those issues which are related to health in any traditional sense from those which are the matrix of society itself. Mental health has viability as a slogan, but its utility for the analysis and solution of problems is at best minimal. As is true of many key terms and phrases in public affairs (and politics), the term "mental health" remains an object of sentiment, not of definition.[9]

Viewing the issues of human behavior from the vantage point of a health-disease model ultimately led to the introduction of epidemiologic models and public health considerations. Such approaches focus upon target conditions (disease) in specific populations rather than individuals, with the conviction that early diagnosis and treatment have limited utility in controlling disease and that what is necessary is intervention in the system to prevent the undesirable state from occurring.[10] As has been amply demon-

[9] See H. D. Lasswell, "The Politics of Mental Health Objectives and Manpower Assets," in *Manpower for Mental Health*, ed. Arnhoff, Rubinstein, and Speisman.
[10] See R. Dubos, *Mirage of Health* (New York: Doubleday & Company, Inc., Anchor Books, 1959); and E. M. Gruenberg, "Application of Control Methods to Mental Illness," *American Journal of Public Health* 47 (1957): 944-52.

strated from the history of medicine, any major changes in social patterns will produce some health effects in the population. Thus, control of the great epidemics and major infectious diseases were brought about not by medical technology or drugs but by changes in sanitation, hygiene, and living standards.[11]

This approach has been proved of tremendous benefit when the undesirable state is a definable pathology and its prevalence and incidence can be assessed. When, however, the target condition is society itself, such considerations and potential correctives transcend matters of health. To the extent that the target conditions are rather vaguely stated, involve moral and legal issues of good and bad, and are imbedded in social values, race, politics, history, and national economic trends, the health aspects are minimal, if not at times altogether irrelevant. In this regard it is essential to recognize that much mental health concern and practice involve not scientific and/or medical findings but, rather, essentially "norm" management or manipulation. Since Albee[12] and Szasz[13] have amply and ably discussed in detail the issues of professionalism, social control, and moral suasion that are maintained by this health-disease model, I need not reiterate these issues here except to state that the politics and economics of mental health are of no small concern. The national expenditures for "mental illness and

[11] *Ibid.*

[12] G. W. Albee, "The Relation of Conceptual Models to Manpower Needs," in *Emergent Approaches to Mental Health Problems*, ed. E. L. Cowen, E. A. Gardner, and M. Zax (New York: Appleton-Century-Crofts, 1967), pp. 63–73; and G. W. Albee, "The Relation of Conceptual Models of Disturbed Behavior to Institutional and Manpower Requirements," in *Manpower for Mental Health*, ed. Arnhoff, Rubinstein, and Speisman.

[13] T. S. Szasz, *The Myth of Mental Illness* (New York: Hoeber-Harper, 1961); and T. S. Szasz, *Law, Liberty and Psychiatry: An Inquiry into the Social Uses of Mental Health Practices* (New York: The Macmillan Company, 1963).

health" are now estimated to be at an annual 20 billion dollar level.[14]

My references to the public health–epidemiologic model should not be construed as criticism of the model per se nor of its broad conceptual applicability to the types of problems we are discussing here. On the contrary, it should be rather obvious by this time that individual corrective approaches produce limited gain: major problems need to be addressed by this total systems approach, and primary prevention is the ideal. In this regard, a medical disease analogue *is* of utility, since no major health problem or condition ever has been brought under control or eliminated by treatment of the already afflicted.[15] Attempts on an individual treatment basis to deal with those people whose problems are viewed as the resultants of social conditions and stresses, as well as with all other "mental health" conditions (intrapsychic conflicts, etc.), show the same prophylactic failure to date.

The widespread acceptance of this preventative mental health approach and the illness concept may lead one to assume that they have been derived from a knowledge base and that direct cause-and-effect relationships, particularly between social factors and later disturbance, have been shown. Unfortunately, this is not the case. While many have questioned the precision or even the existence of such knowledge, one quote here will serve as an illustration of current skepticism:

> One gathers the impression that we have definitive knowledge that poverty produces behavior disorders. Actually such knowledge does not exist yet. We do not know that extreme poverty or extreme affluence increase the risk to develop certain behavior disorders, although this is quite likely. We only know that poverty excludes efficient help or makes such help ineffective because of overwhelming socioeconomic

[14] National Institute of Mental Health, 1967, unpublished data.
[15] See Dubos, *Mirage of Health.*

stresses. At present, we do not possess reliable incidence studies of different behavior disorders, and we have not established correlation between different types of behavior disorders and different types of socioeconomic deprivation.[16]

This was the assessment of current knowledge by one of the pioneer researchers of the relation between social class and mental illness at a recent conference on poverty and mental health. I consider the term "behavior disorders" as still too vague and overly health-flavored. Another eminent social psychiatrist, who rejects the traditional concepts of disease and symptoms when applied to behavior, speaks of a complex continuity between patterns of health and patterns of illness, and proposes a "phenomenal labeling . . . something that might be called *behaviors of psychiatric interest. . . .*[17]

Despite the growing number of publications, conferences, and symposia on social welfare problems, economics, and racial issues which appear under the auspices of the mental health field, there are evidences that a retreat from the all-consuming mental health model may be occurring. Indeed, it was recently suggested that the mental health movement itself has reached an asymptotic level as national concern turns to other compelling issues.[18]

The problems lumped under the heading of "mental health" today and included in the Boston survey obviously go right to the crux of the dilemmas of modern society and involve questions of

[16] F. C. Redlich, "Discussion of Dr. H. Jack Geiger's Paper," in *Poverty and Mental Health,* ed. M. Greenblatt, P. E. Emery, and B. C. Glueck, Jr. Psychiatric Research Report No. 21 (Washington, D. C.: American Psychiatric Association, 1967), pp. 66–67.

[17] A. Leighton, "Is Social Environment a Cause of Psychiatric Disorder?" in *Psychiatric Epidemiology and Mental Health Planning,* ed. R. R. Monroe, G. D. Klee, and E. B. Brody. Psychiatric Research Report No. 22 (Washington, D. C.: American Psychiatric Association, 1967), p. 338.

[18] See Lasswell, "The Politics of Mental Health Objectives and Manpower Assets."

human abilities, skills, values, and even purpose in a confused, fragmented, and rapidly changing society. Even the problems of urban society and living, which are increasingly related to human behavioral conditions, can no longer be dealt with by urban planning and renewal alone, since it has finally been seen that the economic-political-social patterns of America that cause the migration from rural areas must be dealt with to turn the tide.[19] Thus, urban poverty in part stems from rural poverty, and the total country consequently becomes involved.

Until the trend is reversed (and reversal involves overwhelming political and economic upheaval and resistance), the problems will grow. Already 70 per cent of all Americans live on only 1 per cent of the land in 16 major metropolitan areas; and the population implosion in the cities continues. As the Boston West End Urban Renewal Project demonstrated, well-meaning attempts to deal with such urban problems as slum housing can result in *increasing* emotional difficulties for the inhabitants and an increase in "mental health" problems.[20] Other undesirable behavioral effects, however, can be expected to continue as functions of urban overcrowding, the decrease in living space and the overabundance of people,[21] and the adjustment problems of those displaced by automation and industrial upheaval.[22]

Solution, however, becomes increasingly staggering to envision, let alone to accomplish. Consider that the mayor of a typical city may have to deal with over 200 federal agencies in order to obtain the funds needed to deal with his city's problems and that

[19] See J. Fisher, "A Shipload of Doomed Men," *Harpers*, January 1968, pp. 9–12.

[20] See M. Fried, "Grieving for a Lost Home," in *The Urban Condition*, ed. L. J. Duhl (New York: Basic Books, 1963), pp. 151–71.

[21] See F. N. Arnhoff, "Realities and Mental Health Manpower"; and E. T. Hall, *The Hidden Dimension* (New York: Doubleday & Company, Inc., 1966).

[22] See J. Tebbel, "People and Jobs," *Saturday Review*, December 30, 1967, pp. 8–12, 42.

each agency requires specific programs, characteristics, etc.[23] For the most part, however, many urban problems are essentially ungoverned, since their scope now ranges so far and involves so many jurisdictions that coordination goes begging. For example, in order to deal with urban problems in New York City, three states of contiguous, interdependent sprawl, which contain 1,467 distinct, uncoordinated political units, must become involved.[24]

Since necessary corrective or even palliative action requires the broadest social policy actions, it is rather obvious that giving any single factor undue emphasis can produce only the most limited effects or may even prove detrimental to progress. The magnitude of the issues requires the statesmanlike acceptance of basic national realities, epitomized recently by Klarman:

> Outside of the Garden of Eden, following the fall, resources are scarce, so that choices must constantly be made among competing goals and programs. Moreover, whatever society's goals may be, it makes sense to try to attain them at the lowest possible cost through appropriate combination of personnel, equipment, and supplies.[25]

In essence, this is one of the major issues evolving from the mental health characterization of increasingly broad and complex social issues from a very limited perspective: does this particular focus and viewpoint inhibit or facilitate maximum societal return from investment in manpower and resources? Having stated that I see an inhibitory effect resulting from this narrow focus, I would like to borrow a concept from economics to make the point. Following Klarman's realistic dictum on the conservation of resources, the issue resolves itself to a concern for marginal

---

[23] See L. J. Duhl, "What Mental Health Services Are Needed for the Poor," in *Poverty and Mental Health*, ed. Greenblatt, Emery, and Glueck, Jr. Psychiatric Research Report No. 21, pp. 72–78.

[24] See Fisher, "A Shipload of Doomed Men."

[25] H. Klarman, "Economic Aspects of Mental Health Manpower," in *Manpower for Mental Health*, ed. Arnhoff, Rubinstein, and Speisman, p. 67.

costs and benefits—the additional gain from further investment above and beyond current support.

In any given situation, judging by past and current patterns, the addition of more mental health professionals will result in a *slight* increment in total service and care delivery. Needless to say, the specific kinds of services and activities provided will follow from the specific types of personnel added—a point developed extensively by Albee.[26] On the other hand, if we focus on the total system of care and service delivery (the total welfare needs, of which health is but one segment), it becomes evident that other types of services and manpower offer viable alternatives. Addition of other types of personnel and services, for the same incremental cost as the mental health additions, may thus vastly increase care and services to the population.

As a limited example, the primary orientation of psychiatrists in the Boston area toward private practice (average of 50 per cent of total time) is not atypical but rather is the national mode.[27] Consequently, additional psychiatric manpower will produce less net public service increment than the addition of other social-welfare personnel. The same holds true for almost all the traditional mental health professions. The additional (marginal) mental health cost will clearly exceed the benefits when compared to the results that other approaches may give.

The underlying assumption in this total systems approach to health and welfare needs is the firm belief that focus on the emotional aspects of human functioning as a primary cause is too narrow and unrealistic and that in many instances *these aspects*

---

[26] See G. W. Albee, "The Relation of Conceptual Models to Manpower Needs"; and G. W. Albee, "The Relation of Conceptual Models of Disturbed Behavior to Institutional and Manpower Requirements."

[27] See F. N. Arnhoff and B. M. Shriver, *A Study of the Current Status of Mental Health Personnel Supported Under NIMH Training Grants*, Public Health Service Publication No. 1541 (Washington, D. C.: Government Printing Office, 1966).

need never be directly dealt with. The emotional disturbance or disruption is the affective expression of more fundamental problems in adaptation and coping and will disappear if the other facets and needs are dealt with. The kinds of services offered by vocational counseling and rehabilitation, home economics, family planning, mothers' helpers, and the like may be and often are more directly needed.

Viewed, then, in a context of maximum return to the greatest number of people in a system of competing resources, continued inappropriate focus on the health dimension (be it mental health or health in general), will produce limited gain. It will, furthermore, continue inefficiently to consume manpower and capital and to divert attention from the true nature of the conditions involved. Social welfare and provision of corrective assistance need not necessarily include any consideration of illness, disease, or pathology.

I wish to make clear that I am referring to an *inappropriate focus* on, and utilization of, a health-disease orientation to the exclusion of other more productive and socially relevant approaches. Just as it is inappropriate to lump all behavior and social phenomena under the mental health umbrella, so too is it premature to swing to the other extreme and totally reject health-disease considerations. Knowledge does not as yet point to such extremes, despite polemic to the contrary. "Clearly, health cannot be dissociated from any of the factors that influence human welfare and happiness," [28] but in the mental health field its specific relevance remains unknown yet obviously oversubscribed.

Increasingly, it is recommended that the "balkanization" of welfare services be rectified and a unified "one-door" service approach developed: a community service center where the actual nature of the client's needs is assessed on a hierarchy of priorities and where the necessary personnel for implementation

[28] R. Dubos, *Mirage of Health,* p. 178.

of assistance are present or immediately nearby.[29] Until such an approach is taken, individual disciplines, agencies, and points of view will continue to compete for funds and personnel, with political clout determining resolution. In this regard, Ryan notes almost 75 different, independent social work agencies in Boston alone.

Historical analysis meanwhile shows the progressive dilution of the efforts of the traditional mental health professionals as they directly involve themselves in an increasing array of social welfare endeavors based upon theoretically speculative foundations.[30] The initial concern of the mental hygiene movement—the disabling psychoses—remains etiologically enigmatic and relegated to relative neglect. The public health goals of prevention of "disorder" (primary prevention) and prevention of "mild disorder" from becoming worse (secondary prevention) *are* the ultimate goals. While the effects of such efforts to date remain conjectural at best and minimally or inadequately researched, continued efforts directed toward tertiary prevention (reduction of disability) continue to show much promise, and much remains to be done on this level alone.[31]

In view of these varied considerations and complexities, a reassessment of current mental health practice is urgently needed, particularly in reference to poverty and related social issues. Only by such reconsideration and establishment of priorities of responsibility is there any hope for improvement in care and service delivery to all population segments.

The Boston Mental Health Survey should, then, be viewed in its proper perspective—a study of a limited and narrowly focused

[29] See L. J. Duhl, "What Mental Health Services Are Needed for the Poor."

[30] See Arnhoff and Shriver, *A Study of the Current Status of Mental Health Personnel Supported Under NIMH Training Grants.*

[31] See E. M. Gruenberg, "Identifying Cases of Social Breakdown Syndrome," *Milbank Memorial Fund Quarterly* 44 (1966), vol. 1, part 2.

aspect of social welfare services. It is an indictment of American social welfare policies as well as of the current mental health scene. It should be interpreted as such, addressed as such, and no less.

REFERENCES

Albee, G. W. "The Relation of Conceptual Models of Disturbed Behavior to Institutional and Manpower Requirements," in *Manpower for Mental Health,* edited by F. N. Arnhoff, E. A. Rubinstein, and J. C. Speisman. Chicago: Aldine Publishing Company, 1969.

———. "The Relation of Conceptual Models to Manpower Needs," in *Emergent Approaches to Mental Health Problems,* edited by E. L. Cowen, E. A. Gardner, and M. Zax, pp. 63–73. New York: Appleton-Century-Crofts, 1967.

Arnhoff, F. N. "Realities and Mental Health Manpower." *Mental Hygiene 52* (1968): 181–89.

Arnhoff, F. N.; Rubinstein, E. A.; Shriver, B. M.; and Jones, D. R. "The Mental Health Fields: An Overview of Growth and Development," in *Manpower for Mental Health,* edited by F. N. Arnhoff, E. A. Rubinstein, and J. C. Speisman. Chicago: Aldine Publishing Company, 1969.

Arnhoff, F. N., and Shriver, B. M. *A Study of the Current Status of Mental Health Personnel Supported Under NIMH Training Grants.* Public Health Service Publication No. 1541. Washington, D. C.: Government Printing Office, 1966.

Dubos, R. *Mirage of Health.* New York: Doubleday & Company, Inc., Anchor Books, 1959.

Duhl, L. J. "What Mental Health Services Are Needed for the Poor," in *Poverty and Mental Health,* edited by M. Greenblatt, P. E. Emery, and B. C. Glueck, Jr., pp. 72–78. Psychiatric

Research Report No. 21. Washington, D. C.: American Psychiatric Association, 1967.

Fisher, J. "A Shipload of Doomed Men." *Harpers,* January 1968, pp. 9–12.

Fried, M. "Grieving for a Lost Home," in *The Urban Condition,* edited by L. J. Duhl, pp. 151–71. New York: Basic Books, 1963.

Goldhammer, H., and Marshall, A. *Psychosis and Civilization.* Glencoe, Illinois: The Free Press, 1953.

Gruenberg, E. M. "Application of Control Methods to Mental Illness." *American Journal of Public Health* 47 (1957): 944–52.

————. "Identifying Cases of Social Breakdown Syndrome." *Milbank Memorial Fund Quarterly* 44 (1966), vol. 1, part 2.

Hall, E. T. *The Hidden Dimension.* New York: Doubleday & Company, Inc., 1966.

Hollingshead, A. B., and Redlich, F. C. *Social Class and Mental Illness.* New York: John Wiley & Sons, Inc., 1958.

Joint Commission on Mental Illness and Health. *Action for Mental Health.* New York: Basic Books, 1961.

Klarman, H. "Economic Aspects of Mental Health Manpower," in *Manpower for Mental Health,* edited by F. N. Arnhoff, E. A. Rubinstein, and J. C. Speisman. Chicago: Aldine Publishing Company, 1969.

Lasswell, H. D. "The Politics of Mental Health Objectives and Manpower Assets," in *Manpower for Mental Health,* edited by F. N. Arnhoff, E. A. Rubinstein, and J. C. Speisman. Chicago: Aldine Publishing Company, 1969.

Leighton, A. "Is Social Environment a Cause of Psychiatric Disorder?" in *Psychiatric Epidemiology and Mental Health Planning,* edited by R. R. Monroe, G. D. Klee, and E. B. Brody, pp. 337–45. Psychiatric Research Report No. 22. Washington, D. C.: American Psychiatric Association, 1967.

Mencher, S. "Social Trends, Social Policy and Manpower." Paper given at the Institute on Research Approaches to Manpower Problems in Social Welfare Services to Children and Families,

University of Minnesota, Duluth Campus, August 1964. Mimeographed.

National Institute of Mental Health, 1967. Unpublished data.

Redlich, F. C. "Discussion of Dr. H. Jack Geiger's Paper," in *Poverty and Mental Health*, edited by M. Greenblatt, P. E. Emery, and B. C. Glueck, Jr., pp. 66–67. Psychiatric Research Report No. 21. Washington, D. C.: American Psychiatric Association, 1967.

Report of the National Advisory Commission on Health Manpower. Washington, D. C.: Government Printing Office, 1967.

Sanford, N. "The Prevention of Mental Illness," in *Handbook of Clinical Psychology*, edited by B. B. Wolman, pp. 1378–1400. New York: McGraw-Hill, Inc., 1965.

Szasz, T. S. *Law, Liberty and Psychiatry: An Inquiry into the Social Uses of Mental Health Practices.* New York: The Macmillan Company, 1963.

————. *The Myth of Mental Illness.* New York: Hoeber-Harper, 1961.

Tebbel, J. "People and Jobs." *Saturday Review*, December 30, 1967, pp. 8–12, 42.

THE SERVICE NETWORK AS HEURISTIC AND AS FACT

ALFRED J. KAHN

Columbia University School of Social Work

Professionals talk of a service system, a community network, planned intervention. The Boston Mental Health Survey reveals another kind of reality: a service maze, social class as an important determinant of service entitlement and accessibility, professional bias in case disposition, and unpurposive deployment of scarce community resources. It appears that theories of stratification, organization, and communication are as relevant to the improvement of the mental health of large populations as are refinements in intrapsychic dynamics. Behavioral research may increase our ability to treat and cure individuals and families, but we obviously also need planning to cope with problems facing entire populations.

For analytic purposes Dr. Ryan and his colleagues conceptualized the mental health services of Boston and environs as a system or network. In doing so, they were far in advance of the usual local "needs" study or agency survey, for it is obvious that one does not understand the adequacy of any type of social provision without attention to "problems, numbers, people, and places." One must first ask about prevalence and incidence of disturbance

163

and then seek to understand the nature of the channeling system, which ultimately determines who gets where, who is served by whom, and who is allowed to drift unaided or to wander in the spaces and gaps among the demarcated provinces of well-defined agencies and programs.

The notion of a "network" introduces concepts such as input and output. Unlike the individual agency, which may satisfy its sense of responsibility by referring to statistics about interviews conducted or people seen, the network must ask what portion of a problem it addresses and why—*and* whether the total accomplishments of the system match public expectations and the capabilities offered by available knowledge and technology.

The reader is properly warned in the Ryan report that the specific statistics offered probably contain a considerable degree of error, yet the authors are justified in their general critique of the existing network and in the call for planning.

I. Planning a Service Network

As one turns from critique of what exists to projection of improvement, the network concept offers even more specific challenge. One can point to few models; [1] yet some such approach is inevitable, as concern with effective deployment of scarce resources and manpower and with goal-oriented social service increases. Certainly the message of the anti-poverty effort and civil rights revolution of the 1960's is that good intentions are not enough. Social welfare (using the term broadly) is henceforth to be judged by what it delivers and at what cost it delivers. The discussion that follows represents brief consideration of several aspects of the mental health field from a network perspective.

---

[1] For proposals relevant to delinquency and neglect, see Alfred J. Kahn, *Planning Community Services for Children in Trouble* (New York: Columbia University Press, 1963).

BOUNDARIES

In a tentative and very incomplete sense the Boston Mental Health Survey begins to ask about the boundaries of the community mental health field. The question requires far more comprehensive investigation, including experiment and empirical study. From one point of view, people who have emotional difficulties are not reaching the most skilled manpower and are not receiving the optimum treatment regime. But, especially as one departs from the psychoses, the cases now served in the mental health system in Boston, *which is conceptualized as a network for the study purpose but which is not formally organized as one*, face complex layers of social and emotional difficulty which may *or may not* demand psychiatric intervention. There is little or no evidence that they all do better if served in a system dominated by the knowledge and ideology of psychiatry or even medicine. What is obviously needed is a serious effort to determine what types of disturbance are best served under psychiatric-medical leadership and what types are not. The resultant service system should then organize itself to take in those who need its specific expertise and to send out those who do not.

From this perspective, one would refer to a *psychiatry* or *community psychiatry* service system, related to medicine, and not to *community mental health*. The latter is either a social goal —and a vague one at that, heavily colored by cultural and class bias—or the name of a loosely defined social movement, consisting of those who define the "good life" in psychological terms.

A system of boundaries that would place community psychiatry as a service subsystem (or what we prefer to call an "intervention system") within medicine seems to conform to the preliminary criteria for boundaries which we have found workable in a number of sectors in the social field:

——There is major attention to a significant client-patient-citizen-user view of the problem.

——There is major attention to a core of professional-expert knowledge of the problem.

——There is supporting social sanction for the particular conceptualization in the community ethic.

——A defined intervention repertoire exists, is communicable, and is sufficiently different so as to require some unique supporting organization.[2]

In effect, much of the random movement in the Boston service network as conceptualized by Dr. Ryan and his associates relates to the failure of the network to meet these criteria. Case loss would be far smaller were there not the artificial effort to channel people for service in a fashion not supported by sanctions, social definitions, and validated knowledge.

CHANNELING

A network must give major attention to channeling devices and must consider carefully the point at which each case leaves the general helping doorways that offer access to many services and enters a specialized helping channel.

Mental health professionals tend to think of the clergy, teachers, settlement staff, public assistance investigators, and others as what are called "gatekeepers" or "caretakers" in a mental health system. This, however, is a mental-health-centered view of the social scene. That is, these persons are as much the centers of their own social services as psychiatrists are the center of theirs; and the schools, income maintenance agencies, churches, and other institutions are hardly inferior to hospitals or outpatient clinics in their status within the overall social organization—even though many of the individual workers rank below psychiatrists in a prestige system.

The community must organize itself for effective channeling with a view in mind of the main service systems. Its preoccupa-

[2] These criteria are elaborated in Alfred J. Kahn, *Theory and Practice of Social Planning* (New York: Russell Sage Foundation, 1969).

tion should be with organizational devices capable of effecting service accessibility, accountability, case integration, and efficiency. Since professional participants in any service system— whether community psychiatry, education, general (family-child-detached individual) social service, corrections, and so on —tend to a bias in case appraisal and subsequent advice or referral growing out of their particular profession's perspectives, the entry point to any given specific system should be a general all-purpose doorway, not biased in favor of any profession or service system. Thus, it should be as likely that the person who enters the doorway will be advised to apply for social security benefits or job counseling as for family casework or child guidance, if such is his need. The community's gatekeeper should operate with evaluative tools and social perspectives representing a working consensus in a community as to how values, knowledge, resources, and sanction come together with reference to the presenting situation or problem.

There are many notions as to how this is to be accomplished. One approach with much to commend it is a neighborhood-based general information-referral-advice center, adapted from the experience of the British Citizens' Advice Bureaus. There are valid differences of opinion as to whether such centers should be detached or related to multiservice centers; whether they should add policy advocacy or case-advice-referral advocacy; whether they should be public or voluntary, professional or subprofessional in direction. But such a mechanism is needed as a general-purpose doorway to the social service network, "social service" being here defined in its broadest sense to include health, education, income security, housing, recreation, and so on. Such a general-purpose doorway, concerned with rights, benefits, entitlements, and communal resources that are available to all, as well as with diagnostically accessible case services, must obviously have expertise in several senses if it is to be taken seriously. Other essential qualities are the following: an "open-door" atmosphere, considerable range, ability to serve all social classes (stigma-free), confidentiality, nonpartisanship, no sectarian bias, and accountability.[3] But expertise and avoidance of professional bias are the points of departure in implementing the channeling function.

Given geographic, communal, and cultural differences, the function may in some places be assigned to a detached worker, rather than to a staffed center. Whether information center or outpost, it must be locally based, so as to be accessible and adapted to its locale. It must be widely known and as easily found as the post office. Offering services to all social classes, as concerned with resources as with case services, as related to the routines of living as to the crises, it must also avoid an administrative connection, like that found in both public assistance and community psychiatry, which is stigmatizing and closes out some groups.

Such an information-advice-referral service also becomes to the planner a significant "window on the man on the street." It monitors trends, clarifies resource needs, develops policy perspectives, and evaluates new proposals.

At the same time, each specialized agency and resource has reason to reexamine its capacity to admit people easily, to answer questions, to advise, to refer, and to follow through in a fashion suited to its mission, so as to express community concern and decrease random movement. Those people who feel able to do their own case channeling will and should persist in going directly to specialized family, child welfare, public assistance, housing, employment, and similar resources. If the doorways to these services do not assay more than to "sort" inquiries in the light of their *own* functions, selecting what they want and not feeling responsible for the others, the wastage will continue. Perhaps in the long run a network of information centers and outposts will be in a position to service all sub-units and doorway personnel in

[3] See Alfred J. Kahn *et al., Neighborhood Information Centers* (New York: Columbia University School of Social Work, 1966).

specialized agencies with information materials, policy guides, and necessary training. In effect, specialized agencies operate effectively only in the context of consensus about definitions of roles.

ACCOUNTABILITY AND CASE INTEGRATION

Nor does one solve all the problems by alignment of boundaries or improvement of access. Within each system of case services—and case services, after all, are the eventual concern when one deals with the "distressed"—organizational devices are required to assure individualization, persistence, and continuity. He who would create and implement a network must therefore ask about provision for accountability and case integration, as relevant, within the several components of the network.

The "helping" professions have long relied on professional ethics to assure that cases were not dropped or forgotten until service goals were achieved or until there was a deliberate decision that no more could be done and that the community did not need to remain in contact. Similarly, one assumed that adequately trained psychiatrists, social workers, and psychologists would routinely and normally take the necessary initiatives to concert their interventions with others deeply involved in aspects of the family's problems. Now only the naive, the non-readers of studies and journals, the deliberately ignorant can fail to know that organizational and bureaucratic realities generally overcome professional ethics and individual competence. Problems generated by specialization, organizational dynamics, and bureaucratization require organizational solutions. They are, in brief, in the province of administration and planning.

Available experience tells us that there are few true service networks if among the criteria one includes the adequacy of provision for case integration and accountability. Yet the community can hardly claim to be offering a total system of help unless there are included adequate mechanisms for the meshing of the concurrent and sequential services to a family (case integration). Will there be, for a committed delinquent, assurance of continuity from institution to community, with particular reference to schools, responses by adults in various local facilities, and so on? Will the family agency follow through with the family in difficulty, as intended by the referring public assistance worker? And what of the case in which the father is being helped at a veterans' clinic, the total family is on public welfare, one child is in a foster home and one is on probation, and their teachers are concerned about classroom behavior? Who worries about interrelationships and consistency? Who takes the lead in the case?

A variety of administrative devices is employed for case integration, and little is known as to their relative effectiveness under differing circumstances: the intensive worker, the intensive unit, the case coordination committee, the general practitioner. From the social work perspective the evidence mounts of the need for a "general practitioner" role—an agency or a worker who will provide basic counseling and help on an interpersonal level, much as the family doctor does in his field, and who will refer to specialist agencies and services as needed. The general practitioner (the family caseworker before family agencies became specialized) carries case integration responsibility, meshing the services and not giving up the case when it goes to a specialist. He provides continuity over time and between services. Nor does he drop the situation unless the family is prepared to "go it alone," and even then he does not where circumstances place the case in a "protective" category. In short, case integration and accountability are achieved through this one mechanism. Accountability becomes the quality sought in the operation of the system.

II. Interdependence of Networks

Nor can a service network manage alone. If there is a medically guided community psychiatry system (or subsystem within medicine), there must also be a general social service system, not medically controlled, encompassing social services now included under family and child welfare—services to the aged, services to adolescents. And there must also be correctional networks, income maintenance, and other segments of social welfare.

Long experience reveals that no one network is wisely used unless the total system is in balance. For lack of adequate income maintenance, one misuses child welfare; for lack of jobs or job counseling, there may be overemphasis on family casework. The substitute network, being misused, confuses its mission and its intervention specific. Small wonder then, that networks lose their character and, trying to be all things, seldom achieve satisfactory results.

In general, community psychiatry and general social services should be suspect if they offer interpersonal help and intrapsychic counseling in a context in which the basic life needs and services are lacking: jobs, income security programs, housing, health facilities, job counseling, information, day care, homemakers, education. Case services are soundly deployed and have potential for impact only if offered on a solid foundation.

The remaining questions about the social welfare system relate not only to the presence of interdependent services but also to their sufficiency, proximity, accessibility, and quality.

III. Perspectives

A network perspective, then, sharpens the evaluation of social provision. It does even more to guide planning of what is to be; but it holds out difficult requirements. Yet network it must be, for components of social welfare are assigned a broad societal mission. Any given network has functions to fulfill and must organize so as to play its role. All else is rhetoric.

Dr. Ryan suggests "problem-centered" planning as superior to "facility-centered" or "agency-centered" approaches (p. 61). In this, he is obviously correct. Yet even problem-centered perspectives, such as psychiatric illness or delinquency, are not always broad enough. The definition of the priority problem is in itself the declaration of a community policy: to treat or to equalize, to offer therapy or opportunity, to provide a "floor" or to encourage "take-off." Perhaps a "task-centered" perspective is even more helpful—clear and careful consideration of our policies and the development of the several service networks needed, so as to offer the required intervention and help, and then a system to channel cases in a manner which implements our general resolve. Planning, after all, is a normative activity, even when it creates service systems with large scientific and professional apparatus and organization.

RESEARCH DESIGN AND SOCIAL POLICY

❧

MARTIN REIN

Bryn Mawr College
Graduate Department of Social Work and Social Research

The Ryan study, "Distress in the City," presents a thoughtful analysis of an important issue—the distribution of mental health services. A book which includes a series of comments on this study affords an opportunity to explore the kinds of research that are relevant to the development and assessment of social policy in general and specifically the area of mental health. I have chosen to focus my comments on some selected conceptual and methodological issues in policy-oriented research. Let me at the outset assert my conclusions. I believe that research has made a singularly undistinguished contribution to the development of social policy. In short, research has, by and large, failed policy. With the Ryan study as a basis for discussion, let us examine some of the issues which surround this failure.

I. Needs Research and Distributive Research: A Shift of Design

A good deal of policy-oriented research generated by health and welfare councils throughout the United States in the 1940's and 1950's tended, by and large, to be done within a needs-research framework. This type of research attempted to identify the disparity between needs and resources, where resources were defined with reference to the established pattern of professional services and community facilities. Not surprisingly, with unflagging regularity these studies concluded that there was a need for casework, mental health services, group work, or whatever community service was the focus of the inquiry. Such studies were mired in a conceptual confusion from which they could not be rescued. Casework and mental health services are presumably solutions to a problem; however, for any given problem a variety of different programs or interventions can be generated. Thus to start with the intervention and to neglect the problem left the research with a self-contained framework, a circular logic which failed to separate the task from its solutions. Means and ends became blurred, as the service itself came to be regarded as the social aim. And for researchers engaged in evaluative research to insist on the explication of the concrete goals of each service intervention was to present a daunting challenge, which few programs could answer to the researchers' satisfaction. Hence the research either progressed without clarifying the tough question of social purposes or the researcher imposed his goals on the process.

What, after all, are the social objectives of public recreation? To link recreation to a social problem like delinquency would imply that the program might be repudiated if it failed significantly to reduce delinquency rates. But surely individuals would still demand recreation, even if it contributed nothing to the reduction of deviant behavior. This curious situation arises because the framework of problem solving implies that needs are bounded and residual and hence the rendering of adequate services will reduce the need for them. The research model that tried to match needs and resources carried an implicit theory of social provision, which required that services be regarded as self-liquidating. Since many social problems were in turn associated with low income, it was assumed that as incomes rose the need for social programs would decline. But as income rose the cost of welfare programs also expanded. We can account for this as follows: if services are viewed as a response to consumer preferences rather than to problems, they can be seen as amenities which expand choice and enhance the quality and level of living. Accordingly, resources must always fail to meet needs, since needs are indefinitely expansive. Moreover, needs grow rather than decline with increased affluence, as society has the economic capability of responding to an expanding consumer demand for publicly distributed services.

Inadvertently such studies also tended to have an inherent but unrecognized political conservatism, in that they seem at least implicitly to have relied upon a design that reaffirmed the importance of maintaining the form and structure of the established pattern for delivering local social services. This situation occurred because resources were inventoried, not evaluated. Thus these studies supported a type of planning which led to social services aggrandizement in that it sought to expand resources to permit growth of the *prevailing* service pattern. These studies sought, in short, to create a bigger pie without reallocating its sections by function, auspices, or purpose.

There are, of course, other reasons in addition to a limited perspective which account for why prescriptions to relieve social ailments recommended more of the same social medicine. There were also professional commitments which limited vision, political obstacles which impelled planners to avoid conflict, and intellectual problems which made it difficult to develop innovative proposals.

The Ryan study departs radically from these terms of reference. "What is being urged," Ryan unequivocally asserts in his conclusion, "is that evaluation and planning be *problem-centered* rather than *facility-centered* or *agency-centered*" (p. 61). The Ryan study is thus, in effect, an implicit critique of the needs-oriented framework for social policy research. Moreover, the study of mental health services in Boston provides an unusual setting in which to conduct such a critique, since the disparity between resources and services in mental health cannot be regarded as important. Indeed, in metropolitan Boston the

> supply of outpatient psychiatric resources exceeds by over one-third the number generally considered an ideal goal. . . . [The] facts raise some serious questions, first of all about the direction in which solutions should be sought to some [current] problems. It seems quite unrealistic, for example, to think of increased quantities of mental health personnel as a reasonable solution, even if dramatically larger supplies of money and manpower were actually available (p. 56).

If increasing resources offers no solution, then policy must turn to strategies of redistribution. It is clear, then, that Ryan is chiefly concerned with the allocative problem—the pattern of practice and the distribution of personnel. The research findings enable Ryan to highlight the anomalies in the distribution of tasks and resources among agencies and professionals who service those who are in emotional distress.

Most policy-oriented research starts with programmatic conclusions and seeks to support or repudiate these conclusions with convincing data. It is then the objectives of action which form and shape the research design; hence policy preferences are integral to the design. With extreme lucidity Ryan makes explicit his operating value premises when he asserts that it is "necessary to abandon the myth of medical responsibility and to adapt to the fact that, now and in the foreseeable future, most mental health problems involving social disorders—and probably most mental health of poor people—are properly and explicitly the responsibility of nonpsychiatric interests" (p. 55). Thus an examination of the distribution of services permits Ryan to raise policy questions concerning the existing mental health system and its central premise of medical responsibility. Distributive studies tend to be oriented toward social change. They seek to alter the structure and framework on which services are distributed, while needs-resources studies are more oriented toward stasis, tending to seek support for, and expansion of, the established allocative system. In both types of studies researchers may discover facts which nullify their biases and are forced to review their prejudices and operating assumptions. But the more typical pattern is for those who use the findings of the studies to repudiate the research for its methodological weaknesses rather than revise the program in the light of new information. If these observations are valid—if it is useful to think in terms of different types of research frameworks which affect policy—they force attention to the conceptual framework as well as to the facts which might be uncovered. Our strategy must therefore be to consider the research question and the research design in the development of policy.

What factors should influence the research strategy? Freeman has argued that research should select those variables to which the established policy of decision-making systems will respond. Accordingly, the researcher has "an obligation to understand both the organizational needs of these systems and the ways in which research must be structured because of these needs." [1] According to this formulation, it would appear research must respond to, and not challenge, the needs and orientation of the decision-making and -implementing systems of policy. This conception of the role of research as handmaiden to established power can be understood as a strategy to maximize its relevance and hence to enhance its utilization. But the Ryan study does not accept this definition of the task of policy-oriented research; it challenges rather than accepts the premise on which the mental health services' policy and operating systems are based. What effect will

[1] Howard Freeman, "The Strategy of Social Policy Research," *The Social Welfare Forum, 1963* (New York: Columbia University Press, 1963), p. 156.

the fact that research raises social criticism of established power have on utilization of research by that power or by those who wish to challenge power? To examine this question we need to give some consideration to the present state of knowledge about the utilization of sponsored or commissioned research.[2]

II. The Utilization of Research

Sociologists have not in the past addressed a great deal of attention to this problem, and their avoidance of the issue may itself be symptomatic of some diffidence about the extent to which research is used. There has, however, been some work that has sought to specify factors associated with research utilization, which we would like to review briefly. Gouldner believes that in order for research to be effective, it must address itself to the client's real difficulties, which may be different from the requests the client at first presents.[3] This means the researcher must act as a clinician and try to discover what is truly problematic in the situation, rather than act simply as a technician and respond to the client's own formulation of the problem. This emphasis on trying to understand the deeper dynamics of the client system is found in the work of those followers of Kurt Lewin who have done research in industry, the community, and elsewhere.[4] In this

[2] To call policy-oriented research "applied research," as it is the fashion to do, is misleading, because it begs the question of whether the findings of the study will be applied. The term "commissioned research" or "sponsored research" only indicates that someone has called for a study; it leaves open the question of how the research is used, misused, abused, or altogether disregarded. The observations in this discussion are based on an unpublished paper, titled "The Utilization of Commissioned Research" and written by Martin Rein and Robert Weiss.

[3] Alvin W. Gouldner, "Explorations in Applied Social Science," in *Applied Sociology; Opportunities and Problems*, ed. Alvin W. Gouldner, Alvin Ward, and S. M. Miller (New York: The Free Press, 1965), pp. 17–21.

[4] See Kurt Lewin, *Resolving Social Conflicts* (New York: Harper & Brothers, 1948). See especially his discussion of "The Function and Position of Research Within Social Planning and Action," pp. 205–8.

tradition Lippitt searches for common elements in the introduction of planned change into the community, the group, and the individual.[5] In this model the client's difficulties are perceived as a disease, and the researcher is seen as a clinician skilled in diagnosing the malaise, although he is perhaps more skilled in convincing the patient to act on the diagnosis and to overcome his resistance to change. Gouldner sees the need for a clinical sociology "which can aid in mending the rift between the policy maker and social scientist." [6] The important element in this approach is the assumption that research is utilized insofar as the sociologist has been insightful enough to direct his efforts to the key problem of the client system.

Quite another approach sees research as utilized when it gets the proper backing within the client system. Such an approach considers the questions of where the sociologist has entered the organization and essentially how powerful his backing is within it. It is generally thought by those who follow this line of argument that the proper way of entering an organization is with the backing of all relevant groups—the social work professionals as well as the social work executives and the board. Closely related to the issue of support and entry is the nature of the organizational tie between the client and the researcher. The importance of the organizational context for research utilization has been noted by Merton.[7] A generally accepted working hypothesis is that when the organization is the object of the study, utilization of research information increases when the researcher is part of an independent agency. A corollary to this position is that the greater the prestige of the outside agency and the greater

[5] See Ronald Lippitt, Jeanne Watson, and Bruce Westley, *Dynamics of Planned Change* (New York: Harcourt, Brace and Co., 1958); and J. R. Gibb and Ronald Lippitt, issue editors, "Consulting with Groups and Organizations," *Journal of Social Issues* 15, no. 2 (1959).

[6] Gouldner, "Explorations in Applied Social Science," p. 17.

[7] See Robert K. Merton, "The Role of Applied Social Science: A Research Memorandum," *Philosophy of Science* 16, no. 3 (July 1949): 161–81.

the reputation of the researcher, the greater is the likelihood that the information produced will be utilized.

Still a third approach to the question of how best to achieve research utilization considers the way in which research is presented to the client. Here concern is directed to the feedback operation and to the proper ways of enlisting the client's motivation to absorb information and use it in his organizational behavior. Thus some members of the University of Michigan Survey Research Center have concerned themselves not so much with the centrality of the problem they have dealt with or the level on which they have entered the organization as with the extent to which their research information has been incorporated by their client audience and with the development of techniques, especially near-therapeutic group meetings, which maximize the client's response to, and incorporation of, the material.[8]

To summarize, interest in this area has developed around three approaches by which the sociologist may attempt to maximize utilization of his research: first, working on the right problem; second, securing the appropriate relationship to the organization; third, managing the involvement of the client in the process of receiving the information.

Each of these approaches assumes that utilization is dependent in some way on the sociologist—whether he has the right sponsorship and the right relationship to the organization, whether he directs his research toward the right problem, and whether he introduces his results in the proper manner. I would like to suggest an alternative view to these, one which is not original but which has not been given the attention it deserves. This envisions the possibility that research will be used by an

---

[8] See, for example, H. H. Halpert, "Communication as a Basic Tool in Promoting Utilization of Research Findings," *Community Mental Health Journal*, 1966, pp. 231–36; and Robert K. Kahn and Floyd C. Mann, "Uses of Survey Research in Policy Determination," in *Proceedings of Ninth Annual Meeting of Industrial Relations Research Association*, Cleveland, Ohio, December 1956, pp. 256–74.

organization to the extent that it does *not* bear on the central problems of the organization and to the extent that the research avoids implications which deal with the organization's most central dynamics. (Of course, it may be picked up and used selectively in internal power struggles.)

Though this idea may seem paradoxical when stated for organizations, it is very nearly a truism when one concerns oneself with individuals. One would hardly expect to change individual behavior which was deeply motivated and central to the personality simply by communicating information to the individual. Much research and experience supports the view that individuals select information to support their basic commitments and that where they cannot select they distort or deny. Information may help an individual choose means to goals so long as he has no emotional stake in one set of means or another, but information alone is very unlikely to affect goals. The same processes seem to hold true in organizations. Research produces only information and cannot, alone, change the basic direction of organizational behavior. Organizational goals and basic policy or strategies for meeting these goals are molded by values and by the vested interests of key personnel, and these are typically unchangeable by merely announcing information which disputes them. Thus, to increase the likelihood that research findings will be used, researchers must avoid challenging the system's operating premises in any fundamental way and, when possible, should affirm these values by providing a rationale to support their validity. But in such efforts to be useful we surrender the role of social analysis for short-term relevance. Consider the following example.

I recently directed a project in the field of social welfare which was concerned with learning the ways in which certain kinds of child welfare services may be improved.[9] The project was inspired by an agency's desire to become professional and the wish

---

[9] Martin Rein, *The Network of Community Agencies Providing Child Protective Services in Massachusetts* (Boston: Brandeis University Graduate School for Advanced Study in Social Welfare, 1962).

of the top staff to be able to identify themselves with professional service. In writing research findings and recommendations, I wanted to suggest that professionalization was not, at least in this case, appropriate. However, had my report noted that professional workers were not the best for this organization's particular clientele, it seems likely that the organization would then have changed its clientele rather than its professionalizing goal. To avoid this awkward choice, there was always the chance, of course, that the organization would reject the research findings as incompetent and irrelevant or simply ignore and neglect them. It is almost certain that any recommendation that the agency not be professionalized would have been disregarded. So, in an effort to avoid being discounted altogether, I tried to suggest ways in which the agency could continue to do the job that it did in its nonprofessional past after it became professionalized.

But does research that deals with basic organizational problems or that challenges rather than accommodates the predetermined preferences of those who are the subject of the inquiry ever get used? Must we assume that the Ryan study will be disregarded because it searched too deeply and questioned too openly the tenets on which the system rests? I believe there is no need for such a skeptical conclusion. Such research can be used. How can this come about? There are undoubtedly many ways in which criticism can affect policy. Let me comment on one process. I would like here to note the experience of a recent study commissioned by a mental hospital. The hospital asked a sociologist and a psychiatrist to conduct a study with a view toward discovering the therapeutic and untherapeutic effects of the hospital system and the ward atmosphere on its patient population. The report, when written, resulted in almost no changes within the structure of the organization that had commissioned the report. It was felt to be too threatening to the existing individually focused therapeutic ideology and to the organizational position and prestige of present high-level staff. The report suggested a much more sociological, milieu-oriented approach than the strictly psychiatric approach which had previously been the keynote of the organization. The result was a complete failure of the organization to utilize the findings of the research in terms of bringing about changes in its operation. However, what happened subsequently is of great interest. The research report was picked up by the field. It has become something of a classic in its area and has affected thinking in other organizations and among the entering staff and the new executives of these organizations. It has contributed significantly to the changes in the climate within which mental hospitals exist. As a result, it has had a great deal of effect, though not directly on the organization which commissioned the research. The study that I am referring to, of course, is that published as *The Mental Hospital* and authored by Stanton and Schwartz.[10]

I believe that the recommendation in the Ryan study will proably not be fully or even partially implemented in the Boston area, where the study was commissioned. However, its findings will reinforce other studies that have posed similar questions. The cumulative effect of these studies may produce information which will enter the mainstream of thought, become part of the conceptual apparatus of individuals who will staff organizations in the future, and so have a very real impact on organizations of the kind that originally sponsored the research. To illustrate the point, let me briefly review one other study that supports Ryan's conclusions. It may then be useful briefly to review, in the final

[10] Alfred H. Stanton and Morris S. Schwartz, *The Mental Hospital* (New York: Basic Books, 1954). I am indebted to Morris Schwartz for calling my attention to this illuminating example.

I recently did a study of The Planned Parenthood Federation of America that illustrates how the same organization embraced policy recommendations which it earlier had rejected as the political environment changed and national pressure to enhance the organization's effectiveness emerged. For an account of the study see Martin Rein, "Organization for Social Innovation," *Journal of Social Work*, no. 2 (April 1964), pp. 32–41.

section of this essay, the main criticism that may limit the ability to use the findings of these studies of the mental health system.

A framework similar to Ryan's can be found in the research of Elaine Cumming in the city of Syracuse. In her inquiry into the relationship between the distribution of personnel and that of mental health problems Cumming poses a like challenge to the structure of the mental health service system. She studied 275 men over the age of 25 years who had approached various social service agencies for assistance and found that an average of 16 per cent had a previous history of mental hospitalization. The highest rate of previous hospitalization was found among sheltered workshops and charitable services for transients (20 per cent); the prior hospitalization rate for public welfare was somewhat lower (about 15 per cent); while medical clinics and family services had the lowest rates (about 6 per cent). She concluded that

> It appears that the psychotic . . . is allocated or allocates himself to the community services whose workers have the lowest level of training for helping the mentally ill. . . . In all, a principle of allocation on which all agents appear to have a relatively high level of consensus is that the poorer, the more ignorant, and the sicker the patient, the more eligible he is for treatment by the less trained and less professional practitioner.[11]

If there are such inequities in the relationship between distribution of professional skill and problem severity, then, Cumming declares, we must be prepared to face "some vexing questions about the system itself."

Since Ryan in his study does not deal with previously hospitalized individuals but rather with the more diffuse concept of emotional disability, he is unable to make statements regarding the relationship between severity of illness and the distribution of

[11] Elaine Cumming, "Allocation of Care to the Mentally Ill, American Style," in *Organizing for Community Welfare,* ed. Mayer Zald (Chicago: Quadrangle Books, Inc., 1967), pp. 144–45.

professional service. On the other hand, he is able to show convincingly that different gatekeepers have contacts with persons at different income levels who exhibit what the gatekeepers define as emotional disabilities which presumably handicap social functioning. His most important conclusion is that nonpsychiatric personnel and agencies handle by far the highest number of emotionally disabled persons in the city of Boston. The greatest concentration of emotional disability is found in the caseloads of the family doctor and other nonpsychiatric physicians. Like Cumming in her study, Ryan concludes that the distribution of the higher-status professional skills seems to be inversely related to the social and economic situation of individuals who are believed to have symptoms of emotional disability.

Nonpsychiatric personnel try to direct these patients to psychiatric professionals and facilities, which, although adequate by national standards, are nevertheless insufficient to accommodate the estimated 25 per cent of the population who present emotional disabilities. Hence, there is a great deal of motion and activity in which individuals are referred from one part of the social service sector to another; but because of scarcity the process cannot in the end yield services for those who are sent for them. The problem of routing is documented in a special follow-up study of 140 emotionally disturbed individuals who were referred. Ryan notes that only a "small number of clients . . . were counted as having received significant help as a result of the referral process." But even these "were by no means provided with all the services required for the problems with which they were coping" (p. 22).

What inference can be drawn from these suggestive findings? Clearly nonprofessionals work with emotional disabilities, and they rely on a defective referral system, in which few people receive the services for which they are sent. To improve the present referral system would place even greater demands on psychiatric facilities and personnel, yet it seems unreasonable to opt for further growth when Boston's resources already exceed national standards and still appear unable to meet the demands placed upon them. With most communities having dramatically fewer psychiatric resources than Boston, the strategy of expansion cannot seriously be presented as a viable national solution. For Ryan, the direction appears to be the strengthening of the nonpsychiatric system and the weakening of psychiatric control by the breakup of the medical model.

III. Policy Implications of Distribution Research

Whereas the early needs-resource studies proceeded under the implicit assumption that social services could become self-liquidating and that more resources would, in time, reduce the social problems at issue and hence make it possible to bridge the gap between needs and resources, distributional studies proceed under the opposite assumption—namely, that the gap cannot be filled. By calling attention to inequities in the distribution of services by class and by severity of illness, such studies center on the crucial question of the redistribution of resources within the mental health system and the reallocation of resources between it and other systems.

What directions should these changes take? Distributive research, although it dramatizes the need for reallocation much as needs-resource studies documented the need for more resources, does not systematically provide principles on which reallocation of resources to institutions or redistribution of services to individuals may be developed. As we have already discussed, Ryan does offer some hints as to the direction that the reform of the mental health system may take, although in the end he retreats and seems willing to leave the task to a representative planning group, which will include the groups that are most in need of reform. Enough experience is at hand to demonstrate persuasively that faith in local comprehensive planning structures offers no adequate solution for the allocative problems that Ryan has identified.[12] But, rather than pursue the question of the form of planning, I prefer here to give some attention to the substantive choices that are implied in Ryan's interpretation of his findings. For purposes of policy, the most important conclusion Ryan reaches is that more psychiatric personnel and continued reliance on the medical model of responsibility are inappropriate directions to pursue because of the size and the nature of the problem of emotional disability. The author estimates that 25 per cent of the population suffer from emotional disability of such severity as to interfere with their ability to live their lives effectively (p. 9). Presumably a more stringent and precise definition would decrease the size of the population, while a more relaxed one would substantially increase it. But, surprisingly, Ryan's conclusion that one-quarter of the population is emotionally disabled has support in the findings of the Midtown Manhattan survey, an epidemiological study which relied upon six graded categories for the classification of symptom formation. According to this study, only 18.5 per cent of the noninstitutional adult population was found to be "free of significant symptoms of mental pathology," while at the other end of the continuum 23 per cent of the population was classified as "impaired." [13] When studies show that 80 per cent or more of the population show some symptoms of mental pathology, the validity of the concept of pathology must seriously be questioned. The concept of illness is briefly examined later in this essay, but for the moment let us concede that the number of persons suffering from disability appears to be so large that it is altogether unrealistic even to expect that there will be enough fully trained psychiatric personnel to reach all those who

[12] Peter Marris and Martin Rein, *Dilemmas of Social Reform* (New York: Atherton Press, 1967).

[13] Leo Srole *et al.*, *Mental Health in the Metropolis: The Midtown Manhattan Study* (New York: McGraw Hill, Inc., 1962). For a discussion by the author of the credibility of these findings, see pp. 139 ff.

are afflicted with this "illness." Here the argument is clear but inconclusive. Scarcity of personnel requires a more effective system of rationing. But what criteria for rationing should be used? The most skilled personnel could be allocated to those most in need, to those populations which have the highest prevalence of the problem (presumably, low-income groups), or to those who are most capable of using the treatment (presumably, middle-income groups who do not have severe disabilities). Clearly the selection of the principle of rationing—severity of disturbance, prevalence of disturbance, or the ability to benefit from treatment —can either challenge or support the present pattern of distributing services.

The more fundamental assault on the mental health system rests, I think, less on the rationing issue and more on the questions of the nature of the problem of emotional disability, the purpose of treatment, and the appropriate treatment or intervention strategies.

Ryan's definition of emotional disability as "handicap" is quite vague. Presumably, concern with emotional disabilities must include not only the nature of the hurt but also its origins. The concept of emotional disability might be taken to imply that, if a random sample of individuals were placed in the same situation of stress or deprivation, the responses of the healthy individuals would not be so severe as those of the individuals who were emotionally disabled, since the disabled person's response is in terms of personal, rather than situational, factors. Ryan gives an example of a woman whose depression

> is a condition that might seem quite natural in view of what is happening to her. . . . Her emotional disturbance, her marital difficulties, are discovered in a context of serious social disturbance and are only parts of an interlocking system of problems. . . . If she is to receive help at all, she must receive help for her total situation (p. 49).

The problem to be solved seems to be inherently ambiguous, for there is no operational way of distinguishing emotional from situational disability. Perhaps, then, no workable definition can be developed for people who are subjected to overwhelming environmental stress.[14]

In the later part of his report this ambiguity is made even more explicit.

> The direct relationship between social problems and mental health is not only becoming more and more clear; it is increasingly becoming a matter of concern to thoughtful persons in the field. The stressful effects of poverty, poor housing, unemployment, racial discrimination, and inadequate schools are evident in many instances of emotional disturbance (p. 64).

Ryan does not retreat from the policy implications of his analysis that emotional disability may be better understood as a response to environmental stress. Tactfully he poses a hypothetical situation which permits him to suggest that it might be feasible to "induce Boston's mental health professionals as a group to forgo expansion of their own budgets and programs in favor of a drastic upgrading in services and personnel for local departments of public welfare" (p. 54). The implication is clear: emotional disability may better be relieved by intervening from outside of the mental health system.

Perhaps the point can be made more persuasively by considering an example outside the mental health field to illustrate the general argument. Look at the programs designed to improve the physical health of the population in developing societies. It is now

[14] For a discussion of the interrelationship between the social environment and individual personality, see Marc Fried, "Social Problems and Psychopathology," in *Urban America and the Planning of Mental Health Services*, vol. 5, symposium no. 10, Group for the Advancement of Psychiatry, November 1964, pp. 403–46.

reasonably well documented that there may often be a greater payoff in improving the health of a country by improving the nutrition of its inhabitants rather than by expanding the numerical level of health facilities and medical personnel. The first policy leads in the direction of an agriculture policy designed to increase the quantity, quality, and distribution of food. A health goal is pursued by methods outside of the medical care area. This approach contrasts with policies designed to promote symmetry between inputs (medical facilities) and outputs (physical health).

The doctrine that goals in a particular area may be best reached by means outside that area presents a formidable problem everywhere that scarce resources need to be allocated. Consider the difficulty in city government and national government: if, for example, a planner in a city park department is asked what can be done for juvenile delinquency, he'll talk about brightening up the parks, and so on; but there isn't anyone in the city government who will suggest a program outside existing areas or, for that matter, a program overlapping existing areas. Government, then, tends to be conservative in its planning, simply as a consequence of each department's doing the best it can in its own program. On a national scale similar circumstances can have disastrous implications: the military, for example, has peculiar advantages in dealing with Congress—a virtual monopoly on knowledge in a certain area. In order to remedy this sort of situation at any level, a planning department is needed which would have no specific mission but rather would be concerned with the question of whether ultimate goals were being reached. Mental health planning as a model could thus be repudiated and replaced by a social planning unit. But we have not yet resolved the administrative, political, conceptual, and moral issues which such a centralized approach to planning raises.

It is interesting to speculate about other implications that can be drawn from the thesis of dynamic interaction between social deprivation and psychological disruption. In a society where opportunities are truly equalized, failure must be personally damaging, since the individual has only himself to blame for his circumstances. It may also follow that manifestations of emotional disturbance in the poor, even if seemingly equivalent in character to those of the middle class (e.g. hallucinations, delusions, etc.) may not represent so severe a disturbance as the same manifestations in the middle class, where social failure would be far more disruptive; that is, they need not be taken to represent so thoroughgoing a destruction of personality but rather may be considered a more immediate reaction to a stressful environment. We may therefore conclude that treating the poor may yield even better payoff, when an "appropriate" treatment plan is pursued, than treating the middle classes, given the present state of knowledge in psychiatry.[15]

Even if we can agree on a definition of the problem to be solved and the programs and the interventions required, we must clarify the goals of these efforts as well. But once again we encounter formidable difficulties, because

> all psychiatric practice seems to suffer from diffuseness of goals. It aims to restore the patient to mental health, or to restore his ego function, or to reconstitute his personality— terms that can be defined only in such generalities as a sense of 'well being,' or 'maturity,' or, at best, 'adequacy of performance.'[16]

In other words, psychiatry is diffusely concerned with the whole man.

Perhaps the search for specificity of goals may unravel yet another approach for reorganizing the mental health intervention system. The whole man must survive in a fragmented service world, but this may be precisely what is so problematic for those

[15] I am indebted to Dr. Jean Miller, M.D., for this suggestion.
[16] Elaine Cumming, "Allocation of Care to the Mentally Ill, American Style," p. 136.

who have emotional disabilities that handicap their capacity to function. Instead of regarding mental health services as a strategy for *preparing* individuals to function in an unchanged environment, we may need to organize these services to *support* individuals functioning in a changed environment. An example of this shift from preparation to support is found in manpower programs for disadvantaged groups. These programs are moving away from preparation for job placement to the principle of placement first, to be followed by the kind of support that will provide training, health, education, and other services to enable the individual to exploit the opportunities of his changed environment.[17] Hence, one avoids choosing between environmental and personal treatment approaches and attempts to develop a programmatic strategy that disregards these arbitrary boundaries.

Emotional disability can thus be treated by several different strategies: (a) strengthening through additional resources mental health personnel and facilities and reorganizing them so as to reach the low-income group, where presumably such disability is most severely concentrated; (b) reducing disabilities by augmenting the nonclinical social service sectors and the economic sector as well; (c) trying to recombine clinical and nonclinical approaches, on the assumption that situational and personal problems cannot be disentangled and simultaneous intervention in both sectors is required. Other options can obviously be identified as well. Our task here is simply to illustrate the *types* of choices that are open.

Can research help to clarify these allocative issues? Presumably allocative criteria can be developed by examining programs in terms of those which work (effectiveness) and those which iden-

---

[17] For an elaboration of this argument, see "Barriers to Employment of the Disadvantaged," in *Manpower Report of the President* (Washington, D. C.: Government Printing Office, 1968), p. 89. This chapter is based largely on material prepared on contract with the Manpower Administration of the Department of Labor by Martin Rein and S. M. Miller.

tify personal and situational factors that are associated with the problem of emotional disturbance and hence might in some fashion be presumed to contribute to its perpetuation or origin. The first type of question leads to studies of program evaluation and assessment, while the latter type leads both to research that seeks to get at the causes of emotional disturbance and to longitudinal studies that seek to understand the processes by which events become converted into problems. The difference in emphasis is clear: one approach stresses the problem to be solved; the other, the services that are rendered.

The challenge of a policy-oriented inquiry, then, is to develop research that will help to clarify how resources can be allocated and combined so that planning can be "problem-centered rather than facility-centered" (p. 61). This is the challenge presented in the Ryan report.

BOSTON, MINNESOTA[1]

❦

DAVID J. VAIL

Minnesota Department of Public Welfare[2]

I. General Comment

William Ryan's monograph "Distress in the City" should become a classic. In its quiet, understated, superbly documented way it is a *tour de force*. It reminds one of the performance of the master politician who so pervades the middle ground and so persuades the reasonable men who occupy it that no position for contest remains except at the extremes.

A rightist position in this instance would be equivalent to reactionary adherence to the so-called medical model of disease. It can safely be predicted that Ryan's work will call down upon him the old shouts: "Mental illness is an illness like any other illness. It is up to the physicians to determine what is to be done and how to run things." And, "If the system isn't working, the reason is that there is neither a sufficient number of psychiatrists nor strong enough medical control." A leftist position would be equivalent to a total challenge to the humanist values implied here

---

[1] Acknowledgement is made to staff members Richard J. Dethmers for his reading and helpful commentary and J. T. Sarazin for excerpts used in this article.

[2] Medical Director.

and in most of the work now being done in the mental health–mental retardation field.

The framework of values within which moderate men live in late twentieth-century America holds that personal anguish, disruption of family life, anomie, loss of identity, and suffering caused by individuals to themselves or others are problems which must be dealt with. Ryan shows us how these problems are dealt with, for better or worse, in metropolitan Boston in the 1960's.

One could go on praising this work or analyzing the nuances of Ryan's observations. Or one could for the sake of argument take an extreme position and attack at this or that point. I prefer to do neither, and instead will present what I know best—which is the mental health–mental retardation program of Minnesota—against the background of Ryan's ideas and findings. If an accolade is in order, perhaps the most fitting one is to point out that "Distress in the City" and Ryan's other writings have had a pronounced and no doubt lasting impact on program organization in Hennepin County, Minnesota, our largest metropolitan community. More on that later.

Work which we have done in Minnesota since 1962 has led us to postulate several important conditions if the situation that Ryan describes is to be avoided or improved. (1) There must be a rational ordering of the wide range of personal and social problems to be dealt with; these problems Ryan places under the general heading of "emotional disturbance." (2) There must be in a truly comprehensive program a differentiation between the public program, charged with primary responsibility for the problems of public concern, and nonpublic programs that have a broad, flexible, and so to say "self-determining" responsibility for the range of problems that are not necessarily of public concern. (3) There must be a mandated local public agency to carry out the public program at the local level. (4) There must be a local agency which takes responsibility for comprehensive program design, planning, implementation, and evaluation and which also takes into account the entire range of public and nonpublic programs. It is very difficult to see how such an agency could function properly without some statutory base of authority. (5) The state agency must concern itself with the entire range of programs, public and nonpublic. Though the manifestations of this concern vary, it is difficult to see how it could be effectively expressed without some statutorily defined relationship between the state agency and the local agencies in their respective roles of authority and responsibility.

Let us take up these points in turn.

(1) A RATIONAL ORDERING OF PROBLEMS

After several years of study, we evolved the following scheme for ordering the broad range of problems which Ryan calls "emotional disturbance." [3]

I. *Statutorily defined problems.*
A. *Statutorily defined mental problems.* These are problems defined by law. They are of sufficient concern to the public that laws are devised not only to define them but to lay down the ways in which they are to be dealt with. The law furthermore makes government agencies responsible for them and ascribes to these agencies an inescapable accountability for preventing and reducing them. These agencies constitute the province of *public mental health*, and that phrase connotes the same kind of public responsibility and accountability as is found in the public health field generally.

Statutorily defined mental problems in Minnesota, according to a new hospitalization and commitment law inaugurated in 1968, include the following:
1. A mentally ill person (additional variants: a person who is mentally ill and dangerous, a sexual offender, a psychopathic personality).

---

[3] See pages 61–63. He differentiates between "self-identification: the psychiatrist's patient" and "community identification: the hospital patient." He further differentiates various "types of self-identification."

2. A mentally deficient person.
3. An inebriate person.

B. *Mental and emotional aspects of other statutorily defined problems.* This category includes the variety of psychosocial problems that are defined by law and accorded a legal status upon some official event, such as a conviction, adjudication, court ruling, or agency action. Examples are crime, juvenile delinquency, child neglect, dropping out of school, etc.

II. *Culturally defined problems.* Here the culture—the community—judges that "something is wrong" or "something ought to be done." Services may be available and offered, or pressures may be applied to get problematic persons to receive the service. There are, however, no formal legal categories or mechanisms for dealing with the problems. One of the pressures, of course, may be the threat of legal action.

A. *Culturally defined mental problems.* Examples are suicide attempts, mental retardation (differentiated from *mental deficiency*, which is defined statutorily), suspected and diagnosed psychiatric disorders, impulsive and/or hostile behavior, etc.

B. *Mental and emotional aspects of other culturally defined problems.* Examples are marital disharmony, unemployment, underachievement, etc.

III. *Individually defined problems.* Here the individual determines his own status, usually on the basis of some subjective discomfort. (See p. 61).

A. *Individually defined mental problems.* Examples are anxiety, phobias, feelings of inadequacy, etc.

B. *Mental and emotional aspects of other individually defined problems.* Examples are sexual frigidity or impotency, somatic symptoms, work dissatisfactions, child rearing problems, etc.

(2) PUBLIC AND NONPUBLIC PROGRAMS

A truly comprehensive mental health–mental retardation program must concern itself with the entire range of the problems listed above. Obviously such a task is hard work, especially when it comes to making priorities and devising appropriate methodologies.

In the Minnesota scheme the categories of statutorily defined problems (items I-A and I-B in the outline) are the responsibility of the *public* mental health–mental retardation program. This responsibility is represented at the state level by the Department of Public Welfare, at the regional level by the state hospitals for the mentally ill and mentally retarded, and at the county level by the county welfare boards and departments. These agencies have mandated basic responsibilities under Minnesota law.

At the same time, *comprehensive* mental health–mental retardation program responsibility is allocated another way. It rests with the Department of Public Welfare at the state level, to be sure, but thence flows not to county welfare boards but rather to the *community* mental health–mental retardation boards established under the 1957 Minnesota Community Mental Health Services Act.

While the public program is mediated locally by counties, the comprehensive program is mediated by "areas." In Minnesota the area is defined as the county, group of counties, or (in one case) part of a county served by a community mental health center— that is, the area under the jurisdiction of the community mental health–mental retardation board. In some cases, the area and county coincide. This is true in Hennepin County, for example. More often, the area comprises a group of counties. In the state there are 87 counties, sorted into 25 areas, of which 23 have formally organized mental health–mental retardation boards.

There is between the public program and the comprehensive program a difference in the kind of responsibility that is involved. The county welfare board has *direct* responsibility for the public program. The area board, on the other hand, has no direct jurisdiction over the county or over anything else save the mental health center or such other program as it may operate directly.

But it has an encompassing duty to provide total program guidance, design, development, coordination, implementation, and evaluation and to foster resources and expertise for the allocation of available professional skills and services.

A good example of the relationship between the county welfare board and the mental health–mental retardation board is seen in the Minnesota Hospitalization and Commitment Act, which took effect on January 1, 1968. Under Section 10 of this statute, counties must provide "places of temporary hospitalization" (or "public health facilities"), where persons may be detained for "observation, evaluation, diagnosis, treatment, and care" pending commitment hearings. The county welfare board is charged to "assure proper care and treatment" at such facilities. Thus the legal mandate in this instance is clearly related to the public agency (county welfare board) at the local level; but, at the same time, the state looks to the area mental health–mental retardation board to oversee the development and implementation of these programs within its county or group of counties and calls on the area board to be responsible for organizing and/or providing training, consultation, or other services necessary to make this particular feature of the county public mental health–mental retardation program a functioning reality.

(3) MANDATED LOCAL PUBLIC AGENCY

Our studies suggest that the necessity for establishing a local public agency with mandated responsibilities in mental health and mental retardation is poorly recognized, as a general rule, in other places. In Britain the responsibility falls to the local authority, which through local health departments maintains a cadre of "mental welfare officers" to carry it out; in practice, overall continuity of responsibility is often *de facto* carried by the mental hospital. A very highly developed system of local responsibility is found in the Netherlands, where the local authorities (historically for mainly financial reasons) maintain control of each individual case through all phases of service, including inpatient care.

In Minnesota the local mandate rests on the county welfare board. This state of affairs is often surprising to non-Minnesotans. Basing their predilections on the so-called medical model, such persons may express anxiety about the fact that such responsibility is vested in the local welfare, rather than the local health, agency. Such a debate is outside the scope of the present discussion, though our view is that the problems of mental health and mental retardation are at least as closely related to the field of welfare as they are to that of health and that the wisdom of the Minnesota plan will be one day vindicated. Be that as it may, the fact remains that a local mandated responsibility does exist. This is the important point. Given that inescapable accountability is assigned by statute to *some* local agency, it is then of secondary importance whether it is given to a specialized mental health agency, to a health agency, to a welfare board (as in Minnesota), or for that matter to the police. Within the context of the state and local public structure that exists there must be some legislative determination as to where "the buck stops." In this sense the nonprofit agency, while it may be able to exercise domain in program development, in our view simply cannot be expected to possess the legal authority—considering the venerable standards of what goes to make up legal authority—necessary to fulfill the requirements of a mandate for organized public action.

The legal authority of the Minnesota county welfare board in the mental health–mental retardation field is quite extensive. Two examples will suffice. One is the basic statement of powers and duties contained in Minnesota Statute 393.07, Subdivisions 1 and 2 (emphasis added):

> 393.07 POWERS, DUTIES. Subdivision 1. Act as county welfare board.

a. To assist in carrying out the child protection, delinquency prevention, and family assistance responsibilities of the state, the county welfare board shall administer a program of social services and financial assistance to be known as "the public child welfare program." The public child welfare program shall be supervised by the commissioner of public welfare and administered by the county welfare board in accordance with law and with rules and regulations of the commissioner.

b. The purpose of the public child welfare program is to assure protection for, and financial assistance to, children who are confronted with social, physical, or emotional problems requiring such protection and assistance. These problems include, but are not limited to, the following:

(1) *Mental, emotional,* or *physical handicap;*

(2) Illegitimacy, including but not limited to costs of prenatal care, confinement, and other care necessary for the protection of a child who will be illegitimate when born;

(3) Dependency, neglect;

(4) Delinquency;

(5) *Abuse or rejection of a child by its parents;*

(6) Absence of a parent or guardian able and willing to provide needed care and supervision;

(7) *Need of parents for assistance with child rearing problems* or in placing the child in foster care.

c. A county welfare board shall make the services of its public child welfare program available as required by law, by the commissioner, or by the courts and shall cooperate with other agencies, public or private, dealing with the problems of children and their parents as provided in this subdivision.

d. A county welfare board may rent, lease, or purchase property, or in any other way approved by the commissioner contract with individuals or agencies to provide needed facilities for foster care of children. It may purchase services or child care from only duly authorized individuals, agencies, or institutions when in its judgment the needs of a child or his family can best be met in this way.

Subdivision 2. Administration of public welfare. *The county welfare board*, except as provided in Section 393.01, Subdivision 3 and subject to the supervision of the commissioner of public welfare, *shall administer all forms of public welfare for both children and adults, responsibility for which now or hereafter may be imposed on the commissioner of public welfare by law*, including aid to dependent children, old age assistance, aid to the blind, child welfare services, *mental health services*, and other public assistance or public welfare services. The duties of the county welfare board shall be performed in accordance with the standards, rules, and regulations which may be promulgated by the commissioner of public welfare to achieve the purposes intended by law and in order to comply with the requirements of the federal security act in respect to public assistance and child welfare services, so that the state may qualify for grants-in-aid available under that act. The county welfare board shall supervise wards of the commissioner and, when so designated, act as agent of the commissioner of public welfare in the placement of his wards in adoptive homes or in other foster care facilities.[4]

Another example is taken from the Minnesota Hospitalization and Commitment Act, enacted in 1967. Its passage put into law what has been, since 1953, Department of Public Welfare policy. Section 15, Subdivision 12 of the Minnesota Hospitalization and Commitment Act reads as follows:

Prior to the date of discharge, provisional discharge, partial hospitalization, or release of any patient hospitalized under this act, the county welfare board of the county of such patient's residence, in cooperation with the head of the hospital where the patient is hospitalized, the director of the community health center service of said area, and the patient's

---

[4] The statute cited here may be found in the booklet "Public Welfare Laws," issued by the State of Minnesota Department of Public Welfare, 1968, pp. 19–20.

physician, if notified pursuant to Subdivision 14, shall establish a continuing plan of after-care services for such patient, including a plan for medical and psychiatric treatment, nursing care, vocational assistance, and such other aid as the patient shall need. It shall be the duty of such welfare board to supervise and assist such patient in finding employment, suitable shelter, and adequate medical and psychiatric treatment and to aid in his readjustment to the community.[5]

(4) LOCAL COMPREHENSIVE PROGRAM AGENCY

There should exist at the local level some structure—again with authority and responsibility incumbent on it that is clearly spelled out in statute—charged with comprehensive mental health–mental retardation program guidance, design, development, coordination, implementation, and evaluation. While the comprehensive program includes the public program, it includes a great deal more besides. Here is the agency that must assess *all* the available services in the community, both in public and nonpublic sectors.

Minnesota law in 1957 established the community mental health–mental retardation boards, which are permitted to receive grants-in-aid from the Department of Public Welfare in order to establish local programs of various services aimed at "mental illness, mental retardation, and other psychiatric disabilities" (Minnesota Statute 245.61).[6] It is these boards to which the state has assigned the comprehensive program responsibility at the local level.

(5) STATE-LOCAL RELATIONSHIPS

Again, a legal authorization for program development and management is in our view essential. In Minnesota the state agency, the Department of Public Welfare, has the comprehensive responsibility. From here responsibility fans out at the local

[5] "Public Welfare Laws," p. 113.
[6] "Public Welfare Laws," p. 118.

level to the county welfare boards for the public program and to the community mental health–mental retardation boards for the comprehensive program. In both cases a relationship exists between the state and the local agency. In the instance of the county welfare board, the state-local relationship is supervisory. In the instance of the community mental health–mental retardation board the relationship is contractual.[7]

The point is that such clear relationships must exist, or else there can be no coherent structure to the total program.

In Minnesota we regard these principles as axiomatic. Against this background we would regard Ryan's recommendations as being insufficient and weak. It will be recalled that he makes these suggestions:

> There are several different forms which such a planning body could take. It could be established as a permanent part of the existing planning machinery. It could begin its life as a special planning project. It could be attached for administrative purposes to the existing planning agency or the existing voluntary mental health association or to one of the state agencies. It could exist as a newly created independent body (p. 69).

I make these comments in no spirit of criticism against Ryan. In the circumstances he had no choice, it seems to me, but to lay down a series of possibilities for the proper authorities to act on, and I would have done exactly the same. On the basis of Minnesota experience, however, I would hope that the laws pertaining to state and local machinery for mental health–mental retardation programs in Massachusetts could be amended to carry out the principles spelled out above.

A final point, not axiomatic as a rule of operation, but of extreme importance philosophically, can be made. This is that the service model is quite insufficient. That is, the model of the

[7] In this context the state hospitals are construed as a *service* to the area and the county. The relationship between the State Department of Public Welfare and its institutions is a directly administrative one of line authority.

agency or the individual "offering" or "providing" services is inadequate as an answer to the problems that face us. Even the model of a superagency "coordinating services" is in itself inadequate. What is called for is a *program*—that is, a *system*, a cohesive and interrelated organization of objectives that will actively assess the problems, lay down the goals to be attained, and then put together the program elements (that is, the services) that will achieve the goals. A critical issue in this connection is the basic etymology of *program:* it is *something written out ahead of time*—a plan, a set of instructions for what must be done "to get from here to there." Industry, the military, and other disciplines recognize this concept. Why can't we?

II. Metropolitan Minnesota

Minnesota is a very large state geographically, extending roughly 400 miles from north to south and half that in breadth at its narrowest point. It is shaped something like a piece of bread with a large chunk bitten out of the center of one side (east). It has a population estimated in 1968 at around 3.6 million persons. Of these, well over a third live in the two largest counties, Hennepin and Ramsey, and Hennepin (pop. 950,000) contains twice as many people as Ramsey (pop. 470,000). Hennepin and Ramsey Counties contain the Twin Cities, Minneapolis and St. Paul, respectively. The Twin Cities lie southeast of the geographical center of the state. When Minnesotans speak of "the metropolitan area" they mean Hennepin and Ramsey Counties and five additional counties surrounding them.[8]

Counting all the metropolitan areas and other, smaller cities, we find that in 1968 almost exactly half of the state population was

[8] There are, by the U. S. Census Bureau criteria of definitions of "metropolitan area," three additional metropolitan areas in Minnesota: Moorhead and adjacent Fargo, North Dakota; Duluth and adjacent Superior, Wisconsin; and Rochester and its surrounding suburbs in Olmsted County. I make no attempt to discuss these communities in this paper.

urban and half was rural. This poses for mental health–mental retardation and other planning a peculiar problem that must be shared by few other states. It means that at the state level planners must be equally skilled in urban and rural planning. For political, cultural, and economic reasons this situation is obviously a very perplexing and absorbing challenge.

By 1980 it is estimated that about half of the projected population of over four million will reside in the seven-county Twin Cities metropolitan area. This estimate means that it is urgent for the metropolitan community to sort out its various human resource service systems, so that proper planning can take place.

In addition to the axiomatic principles stated earlier concerning the organization of mental health–mental retardation program systems at the state, area, and county levels, we postulate that there must exist legislatively authorized governmental or semi-governmental structures charged with responsibility and authority to coordinate and integrate planning and related efforts. Their responsibility and authority must cover the entire spectrum of planning and program development that is proceeding at the state level, in a host of political subdivisions and human and material resources fields and under a wide variety of public, semipublic, and nonpublic organizations.

Minnesota has made two major strides in this direction. In 1965 the legislature established the State Planning Agency, which is a branch of the governor's office. This agency coordinates planning in all fields within the state departments and their subsidiary and related agencies. The State Planning Agency has been designated as the special state health planning agency as required in the federal P[ublic] L[aw] 89–749 (Comprehensive Health Services Act of 1966).[9]

___

[9] All states, of course, are subject to the influence of the federal legislation and have available to them the considerable benefits that that legislation offers. In this sense, P.L. 89–749 should itself be regarded as a major factor that will have a long-run impact on the problems that Ryan describes.

Minnesota furthermore established in 1967 the Metropolitan Council "in order to coordinate the planning and development of the metropolitan area," comprising the seven metropolitan counties (including Hennepin and Ramsey). This remarkable body is the creature of the state legislature and must report to each legislative session "an explanation of any comprehensive plan" arising in any of the scores of metropolitan political subdivisions that will have an impact on the metropolitan area. It must "prepare and adopt a comprehensive development guide [which] shall *recognize and encompass physical, social, or economic needs of the metropolitan area* and those future developments which will have an impact on the entire area." [10]

Let's face it: unless such instrumentalities are established, how can we hope to establish adequate systems, aimed at the orderly solution of the many human and social problems—including, but obviously not limited to, the mental health–mental retardation field—that face metropolises in modern America? The professionals can't do it, nor can self-assembled groups of well-meaning laymen, nor can piecemeal and time-limited projects; nor can the federal government do it alone. But without these instruments we will end up with the situation once described by Robert Benchley as "citizens bumping into each other carrying trays of hot soup."

Our advice to the mental health and mental retardation professionals and their constituencies is to work through political channels to obtain legislation at state and local levels that will provide the kind of undergirding needed in public law to establish the framework within which orderly change can take place.

In this context one must view with dismay the situation facing the people of Greater Boston. Not only must they contend with the usual economic difficulties of the big city and with deep and often bitter ethnic and religious divisions. Worse, the most serious fault is the low estate of government in those parts and the

[10] Emphasis added. Citations in this paragraph are from Chapter 896, Minnesota Laws of 1967.

virtual guarantee that government agencies established to deal realistically with the problems will sooner or later be shot through with politics of the drearier and more corrupt sort. Though there is not the opportunity to make a case here (Ryan does it well enough), the very profusion of professional staff and training institutions in Boston would very likely constitute a hindrance more than a help in the establishment of an adequate program.

Minnesota, with a proud record of public service and accomplishment and, above all, a tradition of clean and respected government, is in a more fortunate position. To be sure, there are problems and bad ones. But at least a machinery of tremendous potential effectiveness exists to attack the problems systematically.

III. Hennepin County

Hennepin County is a case in point. This is in population the largest of the seven metropolitan counties and indeed the largest in the state, containing about a fourth of all the people in Minnesota. In turn, something over one-half of Hennepin County's population of 950,000 resides in the city of Minneapolis.

Hennepin County has wrestled with the need to produce a viable, comprehensive mental health–mental retardation program. Developments in late 1967 have led to a significant promise for resolution.

An excellent picture of the existing situation in the Twin Cities, and therefore in Hennepin County, is provided in a staff study carried out by J. T. Sarazin [11] and dated December 20, 1967. The study was done in order to support the feasibility of establishing a new (state office) position—that of regional mental health–

[11] Assistant Director, Community Programs Section of the Medical Services Division of the State Department of Public Welfare.

mental retardation program coordinator for the metropolitan area. Sarazin comments as follows:

> The Medical Services Division (of the State Department of Public Welfare) envisions the complex of agencies and institutions as a system. The major problem existing now and for the foreseeable future [is] that most of the personnel and organizations concerned do not share this same view. Instead, they tend to operate quite independently and autonomously, as they have done traditionally.
>
> Most of the professional staff have a clinical and/or hospital orientation, the people involved in mental retardation work tend to have a focus on this problem [mental retardation], and the boards of the agencies tend to see themselves as functioning in an administrative capacity with primary responsibility for fiscal matters. Some boards of the private agencies are only nominal entities and do not meet regularly at all. Most of these individuals and organizations have been very content to operate as they have in the past. They are not certain that they understand or accept the state's demands on them to take on community organization responsibilities, and they do not see themselves as the instruments of social change. . . .
>
> The metropolitan region is much more complex (than other state regions) in size, in its established specialized resources, in its long-standing organizational rivalries and isolation of agencies. While the basic job description of a regional coordinator would be applicable in the Twin Cities, it must be recognized that the greater complexity of this region, containing as it does half of the state's population, will make the job considerably more demanding than it might be in some other parts of the state. Another factor not to be minimized is the degree of complacency on the part of many metropolitan area residents, [who think] that they have such a vast array of services and resources that they have adequately provided for the mental health needs of their fellow citizens. Part of the coordinator's job will be to help educate

these people to see that these specialized resources, while generally of a high quality, could be much more helpful if they were better coordinated as parts of an overall program both for a given county and, in the wider sense, for the entire metropolitan area. Such breadth of vision is not commonplace at this time and will only come very slowly and tediously.[12]

Hennepin County is a one-county area which in 1960 was organized for mental health–mental retardation purposes. Its community mental health–mental retardation board is advisory only, an option allowed by law. The receiver of state grant-in-aid and the legal administrator of the program is the Board of County Commissioners, which is the governing body of the county. The community mental health center is located in the Hennepin County General Hospital, and the psychiatrist-director of the center is the head of the hospital psychiatry department.

The community mental health–mental retardation board for some years was mainly concerned about the operation of the center, a role consistent with the fact that this board also served as the legal advisory board to the hospital. The board more recently came to realize that it has a responsibility for community concern that goes outside the bounds of the center as such.[13]

A plan adopted in 1968 calls for a separate community mental health–mental retardation board which will still be advisory to the Board of County Commissioners but will *not* also serve as the hospital advisory board. More important, the plan calls for a full-time director of the Hennepin County mental health–mental retardation *program*. While entirely free of all direct service or

[12] J. T. Sarazin, official communication, December 20, 1967.

[13] One important event in forcing this realization was the board's effort to designate catchment areas and to design at least on paper a system showing how the Hennepin County Mental Health Center would relate to other (private) inpatient psychiatric services. This effort came about in 1965 in order to fulfill federal requirements under P.L. 88–164 in relation to a construction grant sought by two private hospitals in Minneapolis.

clinical responsibility, he is to have jurisdiction over the program of the center and such other affiliated or related direct-service elements as the board may establish. He is also to be responsible for planning and evaluation, through the establishment of a planning office, of the total mental health–mental retardation program of the county.

The program director will have several critical relationships, and here is the key to the management of the total problem-solving efforts. Administratively he will relate to the Hennepin County administrator [14] and the Board of County Commissioners. In long-range planning he will relate to the mental health–mental retardation board, which is in the Minnesota scheme the area planning agency for mental health and mental retardation. Through the mental health–mental retardation board and the county commissioners he will relate to the Metropolitan Council and thence to the State Planning Agency. Another channel of relationships will be through the State Medical Services Division regional coordinator and thence to the Department of Public Welfare. Another powerful channel leads again from the State Department of Public Welfare to the State Planning Agency. In this system the main avenue for relationship of the official program to the nonpublic sector of private agencies and practitioners will be through the area mental health–mental retardation board.

Staff studies of Ryan's various writings figured very importantly in the official documentation of recommendations to planning bodies in establishing this plan. Thus it is clear that Ryan's ideas have had a pronounced impact on program development in Minnesota.

The Minnesota scheme is possibly complex and certainly imperfect, but it is at least coherent and, we believe, solidly based in law. We think that it will work and that, in any event, it is far

[14] Another legislative breakthrough in 1967 was the authorization of Hennepin County to establish a full-time administrative post analogous to city manager but at the county level.

superior to the kind of confusion that now exists in service-delivery systems in American cities.

Part of the American *ethos* is that government is suspect. The American people tend to believe that nongovernment sponsorship, other things being equal, is superior by far to government sponsorship. The Minnesota proposal is not necessarily opposed to this idea. Nongovernment operation of service components may be preferable. Nongovernment sponsorship of the planning efforts may be preferable, though this is dubious. But in Minnesota we firmly believe that the *system* by which services are delivered and programs are planned should be firmly rooted in law. The law will properly allow a wide variety of options for both service delivery and program planning. But if the services and programs are to be meaningful to the mass of the people, the legal structure and support must be there. For the law is the will of the people and it is only thus that the domestic tranquility, the general welfare, and the blessings of peace will be secured.

WE HAVE
BEEN WARNED!

❀

GEORGE W. ALBEE

Case Western Reserve University

When I first read "Distress in the City" last spring I thought it was the best delineation I had seen of the fundamental problems facing the field of mental health. Now, nearly a year later on re-reading Dr. Ryan's monograph, I am more than ever convinced that my first impression was correct and that the impact of this work may change the whole approach to intervention with disturbed people.

Perhaps "Distress in the City" impressed me so strongly because I had just finished reading a monograph on the mental health problems of Appalachia.[1] This latter report, the product of a conference sponsored by the National Institute of Mental Health, examined carefully the major unmet mental health needs of the people of Appalachia. The conferees came to the conclusion that there are five major groups of people with serious emotional problems demanding intervention for whom little or

[1] U. S. Department of Health, Education and Welfare, *Mental Health in Appalachia: Problems and Prospects in the Central Highlands,* report of a conference at the National Institute of Mental Health, July 13–14, 1964 (Washington, D. C.: Government Printing Office, n.d.).

214 COMMENTARIES ON THE BOSTON REPORT

no help is available anywhere in the hills and hollows of Appalachia. The groups they identified included disturbed children (and
especially those needing intensive residential care), adolescents,
multi-problem families, persons discharged from state mental hospitals, and elderly people. The report of the NIMH conference
suggested that one solution might be "to establish small treatment
units and clinics, operating in different locations at specific times,
or as circuit-riding teams." [2]

When I put down the report on the mental health problems of
Appalachia and took up Dr. Ryan's monograph, I had no idea
what was in store. An hour later I was discovering that the mental
health facilities of Boston (which exceed the wildest dreams of
professional avarice in terms of available psychiatric clinics and
resources) were almost completely neglecting exactly these same
kinds of people. Dr. Ryan points out that there are "five categories of patients . . . frequently mentioned as having little or no
provision made for their care: discharged mental patients, working-class multi-problem families, the aged, adolescents, and children—particularly children in need of residential treatment" (p.
63).

Ryan points out that the required psychiatric facilities do exist
in Boston, and that most of the essential services, with the exception of residential treatment facilities for children, are readily
available in the Boston area. Indeed, Boston itself, with its 250
psychiatrists, is richer in this resource than all of the states of
Appalachia!

I was amazed at the paradox! If a group of conferees in
Washington thinks that the unmet mental health problems of
Appalachia are going to be solved by establishing some clinical
teams, even on horseback, riding from crossroads to crossroads,
or in opening branch offices of state hospitals in the hill counties,

[2] Department of Health, Education and Welfare, *Mental Health in Appalachia*, p. 3.

they had better become familiar with the care-delivery situation in Boston. There, with a cheap system of public transportation and fixed, visible psychiatric clinics and mental health centers, the same categories of people needing help as are found in Appalachia are not getting any help.

It seems quite clear that we may have identified a new social law: the availability of conventional psychiatric resources is completely unrelated to the availability of care for the needs of the poor, particularly for children, adolescents, the aged, disrupted families, and discharged state hospital cases who require follow-up care.

The Joint Commission on Mental Illness and Health (in *Action for Mental Health*, for example) [3] has made the assertion repeatedly that our nation must strive to reach the goal of one psychiatric clinic for every 50,000 people. Although the unhappy manpower realities made this goal seem more a shimmering dream than a potential reality, still it was thought to be the goal toward which we should strive. And, according to this view, on the happy day when we should have reached it, care would at last be available to all.

Ryan's monograph has exploded, perhaps once and for all, the argument that says the roadblock against the delivery of adequate mental health services to the poor is the shortage of professional manpower.

Boston exceeds the hoped-for ratio of one clinic to 50,000 people by a considerable margin. Despite this wealth, practically no care or intervention is available to large groups of the urban poor.

If every city and town in the country were as well supplied with psychiatrists and psychiatric clinics as is Boston, I would expect that the situation Ryan describes would prevail every-

[3] (New York: Basic Books, 1961).

where. We would still be neglecting those who need intervention most—the poor. The secret is finally out. There is no such thing as adequate psychiatric service for the poor!

Ryan's voice is not the only one telling this secret in public. Professor Henry Weihofen of the University of New Mexico School of Law has pointed recently to the double standard of care even in our *public* clinics which, though claiming to be non-discriminatory, somehow manage to give preferential treatment to the middle-class over the lower-class client.

Professor Weihofen says:

> Because psychiatrists understandably prefer "good" patients —those who are sensitive and sophisticated with social and intellectual standards similar to their own—the poor who become patients frequently get inferior treatment, even in the public clinics that purport not to make distinctions between paying and non-paying patients. A recent survey revealed that even a public clinic excluding those able to pay for private psychiatric care still distinguished its patients by social class. Not only were patients from upper social classes accepted for treatment more often, but their treatment was more apt to be given by a senior or more experienced member of the staff.[4]

The recognition of the reality of this double standard of care suggests that the strategy conventionally advocated by manpower experts cannot help but be ineffective. This strategy for years has called for a massive increase in the number of professional mental health people trained with the implicit promise that more manpower would mean care for all. The National Institute of Mental Health has pursued this philosophy with vim. Dr. Stanley Yolles makes cheerful speeches about the gain in professional manpower that has occurred in our nation, largely as a consequence of NIMH training efforts. For example, he says:

[4] H. Weihofen, "Psychiatry for the Poor," *Psychiatric News* 2, no. 10 (1967): 2.

The growth of manpower training in the four core professions is heartening, even though the 1960 baseline was so low
that the increases have not as yet been sufficient to close the
gap between supply and need. All indications point to a continued manpower shortage if the existing rate of training of
professional personnel does not increase. Even so, the 1965
statistics represent an increase of 44 per cent over the 1960
total for psychiatrists, psychologists, social workers, and
nurses. This growth rate is quite spectacular when compared
to a 19 per cent increase over the same five-year period in the
five major health professions of medicine, dentistry, nursing,
environmental health, and health research.[5]

In dramatic contrast to this view are Dr. Ryan's findings, which
should disenchant us all with an approach which implies that our
problems will be solved when our tribes increase.

As a matter of fact, more than half of the total of the nation's
psychiatrists are to be found today in five states. New York,
Pennsylvania, Illinois, California, and Massachusetts claim the
services of the majority of our country's psychiatrists. As these
states are all highly industrialized and urbanized, it seems likely
that comparable patterns of care distribution would be found in
any one of them. It would be interesting to repeat Ryan's study
in another major city in any of these states, if only to satisfy the
scientific purists who want all such surveys cross-validated. I am
confident that the results would be the same. If so, we would have
to decide why other states should undertake the manpower struggle, in the slim hope of increasing their psychiatric resources,
when having an adequate number of psychiatrists makes so little
real difference.

The new miracle cure NIMH is prescribing for the unmet
social needs for care is, of course, the comprehensive community
mental health center. This brick-and-mortar basket, into which

[5] S. Yolles, speech to the American Psychiatric Association, May 11, 1967,
mimeographed.

NIMH is now putting all of its golden eggs, is to be the solution to the terrible state of affairs that exists in the delivery of psychiatric care. In his introduction to the volume on the community mental health center published three years ago by the Joint Information Service of the American Psychiatric Association and the National Association for Mental Health, Walter Barton says, "This program should provide treatment for all persons of all ages and for all types of psychiatric illness. It should be broad enough in concept to meet the requirements of the individual patient at the various stages of his illness." Dr. Barton makes it clear that he is not talking about the privileged few but about everyone. He says that this "program . . . provides total mental health services to meet the total needs of the community." [6]

The centers program will be a failure, probably for the same reasons that the state mental hospitals are a failure. The chronic problem with which our field must deal is the delivery of intervention and care to the people who need it most—the poor. But because of the intransigent stand of American medicine, which is in opposition to tax-supported medical intervention, the centers rarely will be built and staffed as tax-supported facilities; and yet public facilities are the only kind that can serve the poor. Rather, as is already happening, the centers will be grafted onto those general hospitals with existing psychiatric units. This solution will be extremely advantageous to the private psychiatrists who have bed privileges in these general hospitals. Because the ground rules are drawn in such a way that 90 per cent of the new beds constructed in general hospitals may be closed to the indigent but will be available to the middle-class private psychiatric patient with Blue Cross or other hospitalization insurance and with the financial resources to pay for his private psychiatric care in the

---

[6] Walter Barton, Introduction to *The Community Mental Health Center: An Analysis of Existing Models,* by R. Glasscote *et al.* (Washington, D. C.: The Joint Information Service of the American Psychiatric Association and the National Association for Mental Health, 1964).

general hospital, the centers will simply expand the resources available to those now claiming most of the care anyway.

This situation cries out to heaven for justice. Well-to-do people can obtain reasonably good psychiatric care, within the limits of available knowledge, and they assume that care is available for all. This "let-them-eat-cake" attitude reflects the characteristically myopic view of the great American white middle class and its lack of awareness of the netherworld of the city.

The decisions leading to a program of construction of comprehensive mental health centers resulting from an alliance between psychiatry and citizens' mental health organizations are remarkably similar to those that have prevailed in the field of mental retardation research. The late President Kennedy convinced the Congress that large sums of federal money should be made available for research in the field of mental retardation, and funds have been appropriated for the construction of a number of large research centers. But these research centers have turned out to be almost exclusively in biomedical settings and to be oriented toward expensive, highly technical research into the relatively rare and esoteric forms of severe retardation, which involve something less than ten per cent of all the retarded. The overwhelming majority of the retarded—those normally healthy children who have IQ's ranging from 50 to 85 and who constitute *almost 15 per cent of the total population*—is almost entirely neglected by the bold new federal research support program. Why? For the same kinds of reasons that the mentally disordered poor are neglected. No one is organized to speak for them. When well-to-do upper-middle-class parents have a retarded child, the condition most usually arises out of exogenous or structural causes, such as infections, birth damage, or physical anomalies. These parents, joining together with others like themselves, form citizens' groups that lobby effectively for more biomedical research into discovering the causes of defects like the ones their own children suffer. On the other hand, parents of garden-variety, "normally" retarded children do not become members of these citizens' groups; they are not organized, they have no spokesmen, and indeed they may have little sophisticated awareness or knowledge about the extent of their childrens' intellectual deficiencies.

In both these new federally supported programs scarce and expensive professional time for both research and service will be available for the few but not for the many. Ryan says that for many "there is no place, there are no people, there is no time" (p. 12).

Ryan also explodes the widespread myth that psychiatrists in private practice are treating and making more effective the gate-keepers, the influential people in the community, who are having a beneficial "ripple effect" as a result of their increased effectiveness. Reality turns out to be quite different. The typical psychiatric client was found by his survey to be a young, white, upper-middle-class, college-educated female. In nearly half the cases she had had previous psychiatric care. Her symptoms were predominantly anxiety and depression. Hardly a gatekeeper, in the usual sense!

It is instructive to learn from Ryan's factual reporting that it is the social casework agencies and the settlement houses, together with the clergy and non-psychiatric physicians, who are the major care-givers even in Psychiatryland!

Half of Boston's emotionally disturbed citizens receive no intervention from any source. Casework agencies intervene actively with twice as many people as do psychiatric clinics. Perhaps the most eye-opening finding is the fact that settlement houses and similar agencies care for twice as many disturbed children as do the child psychiatry clinics, despite the widespread national visibility of Boston as a center and leader in the child psychiatry field. Clergymen in Boston work with more disturbed people than do psychiatrists.

Do we need more evidence of the bankruptcy of our present model before we are willing to face the reality that the estab-

lished system does not work, that the Emperor has no clothes, and
that the inordinate amount of money we pour into the training
and support of mental health professionals and clinics is mostly
money down a golden drain?

Over and over again we are told that it is the poor—poor
children, poor aged persons, poor teenagers, poor ADC mothers,
and poor discharged state hospital victims (described by Ryan on
being sent to the hospital as "poor and no longer young, . . .
often living alone, isolated from any social connections" p. 19).
—for whom practically no care is available.

Ryan, in his quiet, almost genteel style, makes a modest proposal which, once understood, is so audacious that in another age
he would have been tried for heresy and boiled in oil. He really
nails it to the door! He suggests that, if Boston's mental health
professionals as a group were to recognize that some

> patterns of social and emotional pathology . . . may very
> appropriately be removed from the province of accepted
> psychiatric responsibility, . . . [they] might, as a highly
> hypothetical example, [be induced] to forgo expansion of
> their own budgets and programs in favor of a drastic upgrad-
> ing in services and personnel for local departments of public
> welfare (p. 54).

Former H.E.W. Secretary John Gardner has put it to us forth-
rightly:

> I believe we are now in a situation in which the gravest con-
> sequences for this nation will ensue if we fail to act decisively
> on the problems of the cities, poverty and discrimination.
> The human misery in the ghettos is not a figment of the
> imagination. It can be read in the statistics on infant mortal-
> ity, in the crime statistics, in the unemployment figures, in
> the data on educational retardation. We must deal respon-
> sively and not punitively with human need. . . . We are in
> deep trouble as a people. And history is not going to deal

kindly with a rich nation that will not tax itself to cure its miseries.[7]

The image that keeps coming to my mind when I think about our mental health activities is the brightly lit German night club in the Broadway musical *Cabaret*, where in an atmosphere of complete artificiality and phoniness a group of professional call-girls spend their time telephoning each other and their clients, while outside there grows the unmistakable sound of approaching horror.

REFERENCES

Barton, Walter. Introduction to *The Community Mental Health Center: An Analysis of Existing Models*, edited by Raymond Glasscote, H. M. Forstenzer, and A. R. Foley. Washington, D. C.: The Joint Information Service of the American Psychiatric Association and the National Association for Mental Health, 1964.

Gardner, John. "No Easy Victories." Speech given to the American Statistical Association, December 27, 1967. Mimeographed.

Joint Commission on Mental Illness and Health. *Action for Mental Health*. New York: Basic Books, 1961.

U. S. Department of Health, Education and Welfare. *Mental Health in Appalachia: Problems and Prospects in the Central Highlands*. Report of a conference at the National Institute of Mental Health, July 13–14, 1964. Washington, D. C.: Government Printing Office, n.d.

Weihofen, Henry. "Psychiatry for the Poor," *Psychiatric News* 2, no. 10 (1967): 2.

Yolles, Stanley. Speech given to the American Psychiatric Association, May 11, 1967. Mimeographed.

---

[7] John Gardner, "No Easy Victories," speech given to the American Statistical Association, December 27, 1967. Mimeographed.

III
A NEW
MENTAL HEALTH
AGENDA

❦

WILLIAM RYAN

INTRODUCTION

Except in the realm of fantasy and daydream, one is rarely given the chance to go over again an action of the past. I find it an unusual experience to look back at the work of the Boston Mental Health Survey and at the summary report I wrote five years ago and to be able to comment on it in print. It is as if, during a conference, one were able to be the discussant of one's own paper. To have, in addition, the benefits of the many excellent insights, extensions, elaborations, and analyses to be found in Part Two of this book makes the experience even more remarkable.

Let me at this point forecast what I will be putting down on the following pages. I will not, except incidentally, comment directly on the original report. My initial concern will be to respond to the many issues and problems that have been raised by the commentators. As I see it, these fall into four categories. First, there are program issues with respect to how services should be organized and staffed and what priorities should be established in making these kinds of decisions. Such questions are particularly prominent in the essays by Levinson, Albee, Rowland, Duhl, and Amrine. A second group of issues can be grouped together under the topic of planning. Here the relevant essays are those contributed by Kahn, Vail, Rein, and, again, Levinson. A third set of problems revolves around a number of more general policy questions raised by Duhl, Albee, Rein, and others. The final set of issues relates to the question of how we conceptualize mental health problems and mental health programs. Arnhoff's exceptionally thoughtful commentary bears most directly on this issue, but those by Kahn, Levinson, Duhl, and Albee are also significant.

My plan, after commenting on these four sets of issues, is to devote some space to a discussion of the disease model in mental health services. This particular problem, which was raised by a number of the discussants, is becoming more and more central as we push along the mental health enterprise in this country. A final section of Part Three will address some of my own concerns about the way the relationship between poverty and emotional disorder is being treated theoretically and practically. In particular, I plan to focus attention on what I perceive to be some of the dangers inherent in the formulations being put forth in the growing literature on this topic.

COMMENTARY ON THE COMMENTARY

※

I. Program Issues

Let me plunge now directly into a discussion of some of the serious and often knotty issues that have been raised by the nine excellent essays you have just finished reading, beginning with two kinds of program issues: the performance of the mental health center and the question of prevention.

THE MENTAL HEALTH CENTER

Programming for mental health services is more and more focusing on, and being contained within, the new concept of the community mental health center. It should perhaps be no surprise to us that this is so. The pumping of new money into a field necessarily shapes the development of that field and the big new money in mental health comes in the form of construction grants and staffing grants from the federal government, together with matching and supporting funds from local tax and voluntary sources. It is time to start asking whether the mental health center, as it is now rather rigidly conceived, is a sufficient response to what we know about the nature and extent of human problems relating to emotional disorder.

The mental health center was invented to solve many of the kinds of problems that were identified in the Boston survey and in similar studies elsewhere and which have been underlined so vividly by the contributors to this book. It is designed as a solution, for example, to the problem of separation of patients from their communities, which has been shown to be so harmful. It is a solution to the problem of fragmented and incomplete services through the notion of comprehensiveness of program and continuity of care. And it is, perhaps most important, a solution to the problem of selectivity in the delivery of services—i.e., the exclusion of the poor, of minority groups, and of other segments of the population from access to mental health services. That is, mental health centers have an explicit commitment to provide coverage to the given populations within their catchment areas for the mental health problems that are relevant to those populations. These three "C's" of community mental health—comprehensiveness, coverage, and community—must be considered in some detail.

Comprehensiveness.

Let us begin by asking ourselves: "What do we mean by the term 'comprehensive services'?" In one sense, the answer has already been defined to a perilously exact degree by the federal regulations which list the five necessary and five desirable service components that are considered to make up a comprehensive program. This is a legitimate way of defining the term, but it does have some defects: in defining comprehensiveness in terms of a range of services, we tie ourselves in large measure to the past, in that we are able to include only those kinds of practices and procedures that have attained a name and an established status. In this sense, comprehensiveness means only that all of the different kinds of services that have so far been devised by psychiatric practitioners should be included in any new program. Unfortunately such a definition often leads to a situation where "maximum" and "minimum" are defined in precisely the same way. That is, we are constrained to provide the five basic services but often are at the same time constrained not to provide very much else.

We also in this way bind ourselves very closely to a medical model. We talk about inpatient and outpatient programs, rehabilitation programs, partial hospitalization, etc. This focus derives from, and reinforces, a definition of the emotionally disturbed person as a *patient*—that is, as an ill person with a need for medical treatment. We also tie ourselves in some measure to the idea of treatment directed primarily to the more severely disturbed. The only real escape hatch in the regulations governing programs of mental health centers is the category of consultation and education, which is fairly broad and undefined and would cover, for example, preventive programs.

I would suggest that there is another and perhaps more meaningful way of thinking about comprehensiveness, which is to focus not on the services we have available but on the needs of the emotionally disturbed person. In this sense, then, comprehensiveness would be achieved when a mental health program was broad enough to give meaningful help to all persons with mental problems. This kind of issue becomes most clear and relevant when we are confronted with what is usually called a "multi-problem family." Such a family might have a set of problems that include unemployment, alcoholism, poor housing, child-neglect, and depression in the mother. The tangle of causes and effects among these various kinds of problems is very difficult to sort out: is the alcoholism, for example, a symptom of depression or a reaction to the unemployment? Is the child-neglect a result of the alcoholism or of the depression or of both? Finally, and most important to this discussion, which of the ten proposed services that constitute a comprehensive mental health center program are applicable to such a family in a manner that is uniquely tailored to their needs? Why, for example, would treatment in a day hospital or outpatient therapy or rehabilitation services be particularly suited to some or all of the members of this family as against some or all the members of some other family that has a much more focused and bounded problem?

As we begin to move away from our offices and the walls of the buildings we work in, and as we start to make more use of members of the population we are contracting to serve (the so-called indigenous nonprofessionals), we find that we are being forced more and more to deal with these kinds of problem complexes and that most of the activities we are starting to engage in—most of what we might call "services"—cannot readily be fitted into any one of the program elements that we have become familiar with. Community workers operating out of mental health centers find themselves dealing with housing problems, with employment problems, and with welfare problems; and they are finding out that it is often more relevant to ask a client "Are the people who live in your building organized in a tenants' council?" than to ask about the toilet-training of the children.

I am suggesting that comprehensiveness of program must in the long run be defined primarily in terms of the kinds of problems that emotionally disturbed persons have. It was perfectly appropriate to make a first approximation of what this range might be by specifying the ten mental health center services. But it would be highly unfortunate if the notion of comprehensiveness were to be frozen in the form of that first approximation. The ultimate question is "Have we devised and put into practice the kinds of services that are appropriate to, and proportionate to, the total set of problems that are presented to us?" Hopefully, our asking this question would mean that we are going to devise new kinds of services before we are content to tell ourselves that we are providing a comprehensive program.

Coverage

The second question raised by the advent of the community mental health center is that of coverage, in some ways the most revolutionary element in the whole idea of community service. Up until the last few years the concept of coverage has never been central in the minds of those who think about mental health services, although of course most states make a partial commitment to provide coverage for one particular type of mental health problem—the blatantly psychotic individual who is completely intolerable to the community. We do have a commitment to remove such individuals from the streets and give them treatment somewhere. Beyond this, our society has never agreed that it should give some kind of help to everyone with mental illness or emotional disturbance.

This lack contrasts with our commitment to coverage in other areas of human service, such as financial assistance, child placement, and medical care in acute emergency situations. A man who is struck by an automobile or has a heart attack will ordinarily be brought to a hospital somewhere nearby and will be given treatment, no matter who he is or whether he can pay all, or any part of, the cost. Similarly, if a child is severely neglected or deprived of parental care, our society is committed to the task of finding a home for the child to stay in and a family to take care of him. And, if a family is without money, we rarely permit them actually to starve to death. Through public—or occasionally private—resources, we provide some minimal amount of financial assistance.

In the mental health field such a commitment to coverage has never been made, but the rhetoric of the community mental health center implies that we are about to do so. Such an intention would have enormous implications. Consider what it would mean in terms of numbers. It is generally accepted that only a very small minority of the emotionally disturbed are provided with any sort of services in psychiatric settings. A commitment to coverage could well mean an increase of five- or tenfold in the provision of such services. As has been pointed out over and over again, we are unable or unwilling to increase our financial investment in mental health by a factor of five or ten or twenty. And even if we were ready to do so, we do not have and probably never will have enough skilled manpower to make use of such an investment.

Still, we have begun to promise to care for vastly larger numbers of the disturbed. How are we to do it? It seems clear that a number of avenues must be explored, including a drastic increase in productivity of psychiatric services and a formal systematic increase in the mental health role of nonpsychiatric agencies and individuals.

The latter kind of development could present very painful choices for those in the mental health field, for, if we are to expect nonpsychiatric agencies to increase their mental health role, it is only logical to expect that they must also increase their financial resources, their staff resources, and their training resources. This could conceivably mean that we would find ourselves, if we follow our logic to the end, supporting an increase in the budget of other agencies and a ceiling on the budget of our own, psychiatric, agencies.

All of this, also, points to the need for coordination and integration of services and a greater emphasis on continuity of care —which translates, in very simple terms, to the need for increased planning.

One would suppose—incorrectly—that it is hardly necessary to underline another aspect of the commitment to coverage—that of correcting the discriminatory effect of past practices, which, by providing fewer and lower quality services to the poor and to the black, have had precisely the opposite effect one would expect from a coverage policy.

Community

The third issue raised by the federal community mental health centers program is semantic: what do we mean by the term "community" itself? To some, the definition has been a purely geographic one; to others the word has a larger connotation. The simple idea of making services more physically accessible, closer to home, has been the core meaning of much activity that has paraded under the banner of community mental health. This idea represents the purely geographical definition, and I for one am inclined to suspect those who cling to it of disingenuousness. The other sense of the term connotes more. It implies that we are intending to connect mental health services into the life of the community. In order to accomplish this, it is necessary to make more inclusive the range of those involved in decision-making about programs and priorities.

When we talk about increasing responsibility for mental health at the local level and about increasing the amount of citizen participation in decentralized decision-making, many people start to get very nervous about what they call politics. The answer to the question "How are we to keep politics out of mental health?" is very simple. We will *not* keep politics out of mental health, and under almost every arrangement now in existence we *do* not keep politics out of mental health. We all engage in political activity in the form of lobbying for legislation or for budgets, and this is certainly putting politics into mental health. In addition, in many states hundreds and often thousands of jobs within the institutions of the mental health authority are, to the practical politician, a major source of patronage. It is idle to pretend that a public agency at the state level, at the local level, or at the federal level can in any sense be isolated from politics. We must face the fact that the participation of citizens in decision-making and in policy-setting *is* politics. That's what politics is all about. If we were to exclude local interests, as is the case in some states, we would be making an equally political decision. The very essence of politics is decision-making about public action, about public policy. Why should mental health be excluded from a process by which we shape policy about education, public assistance, road construction, zoning, police protection, and all the other functions of the community.

One man's politics is another man's democracy.

These, then, are some of the central issues raised by the federal program to support the building and staffing of mental health centers. How they are resolved remains to be seen, but that they are serious and pressing can hardly be denied.

PREVENTION

One can find throughout the foregoing essays and throughout much of the literature in the mental health field three different points of view about the problem of prevention in mental health which emphasize, respectively, education, communication, and social action. We are most familiar with the educational approach, since we have tended to use this most often in the past. We have developed popular literature around child-rearing issues. We have conducted workshops and seminars for parents and for those we have chosen to call "caretakers," and we have made some efforts to develop approaches toward mass educational activities. Loyd Rowland's tracing of the history of the *Pierre the Pelican* series suggests that these efforts have had substantial impact. They are appreciated by the recipients and they apparently lead to some significant changes in the attitudes and in the behavior of particular parents.

The other two areas—communication and social action—have not had very substantial investments of time and energy. Our experience with them is extremely limited. Personally, I have developed some hunches—that may be no more than prejudices —about these questions. We have some substantial evidence at this point that emotional disorder, at least that which is of a temporary nature, is closely related to social injustice as it is reflected in such problems as slum housing, unemployment, and racial discrimination. In the last few years those of us in the mental health field have begun to turn our attention to these issues and, in a few cases, even to venture into these fields in a programmatic way. Problems of welfare, problems of housing, problems of police practices have more and more come to our attention. There is a crucial issue to be faced as we move into these areas—the issue of attitude towards advocacy. On the one hand, there are those who feel that the basic issue is one of communication and the improvement of communication between dominant and subordinate groups. Thus we see efforts to provide sensitivity training groups made up of police officers and ghetto residents. We see efforts to improve communication between school administrators and teachers on the one hand and parents and students on the other hand. These efforts are based fundamentally on the assumption that the major difficulty in poverty areas and ghettos and in the whole field of urban problems is one of misunderstanding, and on a further assumption that, since mental health professionals are experts in the area of communication and misunderstanding, a suitable role for them is to try to reduce the volume of misinformation and to improve communication. Another way of looking at the same phenomena is to see that urban problems are in the main a reflection of injustice, inequality, and oppression. Assuming this to be so, one could conclude that such problems can best be alleviated by social change. If one comes to such a conclusion, then one is propelled toward the role of advocate and ally of the poor, the black, and the exploited. In addition, one is guided in the area of program development toward the realm of social action. The choices of verbs and adjectives I have made in the previous sentences surely reveal the fact that I find myself on the side of those who favor an advocacy position.

For example, one of the activities we have developed at the Connecticut Mental Health Center has been the assignment of a community organization team to work with welfare recipients on problems that the recipients have identified as being of major concern to them. In the course of working with the welfare mothers, our community organization team quickly moved into an advocacy position, helped to facilitate the organization of a welfare rights group, and worked closely with the mothers in their confrontation with the Welfare Department about such issues as meeting the department's own standards for clothing for children. In the course of this activity, a number of the mothers were arrested—in what seemed to us a highly arbitrary and illegal manner—and our workers, fortunately, had the courage to stand with the mothers they had been working with, and they were also arrested. This incident led to a great deal of controversy and criticism of the Connecticut Mental Health Center, but the core and center of the issue is what happened to the mothers. Those of us who have been close to this action have observed a dramatic increase in energy, in self-esteem, in self-confidence, and in willingness to take an active role in trying to influence what happens to them. This seems to us to be an increment in mental health, and we believe that the activities of our workers in taking this role have been consonant with a mental health orientation.

The question, then, is not only how much we will begin to turn some of our energies into the area of prevention, as opposed to the area of treatment, but also what forms these energies will take. Educational and family life training activities obviously must continue. They have a clearly demonstrated effect and are important, but at the same time I would suggest that as mental health professionals and as persons interested in mental health we must start moving into the area of social problems and social injustice and begin to take a larger and larger role in social action efforts to bring about social change.

II. Planning Issues

Some of the most substantial issues raised, particularly those discussed by Kahn and Vail, have to do with planning.

In my view, urban mental health planning today must be based on certain imperatives. We must, for example, accommodate the growing importance of the public sector and the public agency.

We must recognize the interdependence of the purely psychiatric agency and other agencies with somewhat different missions in the health and welfare system. We must pay close attention to the question of the boundaries between the mental health system and other service systems, and we must concern ourselves with the question of accountability and its implications.

Having recently concluded a preliminary study of mental health planning in metropolitan areas throughout the country, I have certain clearly defined opinions or, if you will, prejudices. It seems clear, for example, that there are certain trends, largely of a historical nature, to which we must adapt. These trends have a substantial bearing on how mental health services are planned and administered, since they reflect shifts in the way human services in general are thought about and carried out.

Close observation of developments in the delivery of human services will disclose certain clear historical trends. Whether we choose a long term perspective—such as the comparison of the Poor Laws of Elizabethan England with the legislative structure of the modern welfare state—or a short term perspective—such as a comparison of American social welfare thought in the New Deal days of the 1930's with analogous ideas in the 1960's—we find that the trend lines point to a similar progression or developmental line that reflects a more or less unitary underlying dimension.

The anchor points, the positions *from* which and *to* which these trend lines seem to be moving, can be defined in several different ways. For example, there is a movement from private arrangements to public arrangements; there is a movement from the voluntary to the legislated; there is a trend from programs directed to specially defined groups to those designed for much larger groups or even for the community at large; there is a trend from a narrow exclusive base of participation in decision-making to a broader, more inclusive base; there is a movement from the reparative or the remedial to the preventive or promotive; and there is a trend from locally based to nationally based arrangements.

Let me give a few illustrations. First, private to public. At one time, the problem of what used to be called pauperism was a matter for private interests to take care of—philanthropic citizens, neighbors, the institutions of the church and, later, charitable organizations. Now the problem is redefined as one of income maintenance and is attended to largely through mechanisms of public assistance. In the specific field of mental health there has also been a steady expansion of the public role, first in the publicly operated lunatic asylums or state hospitals, later in the area of generalized public support of training, research, and demonstrations, and, still later, in the introduction of publicly supported outpatient and community services. The trend is clearly from the private domain to the public arena.

Second, we see the movement from voluntary to planned and legislated arrangements. At one time, the provision of human services and the meeting of human needs was in the realm of charity, which is, by definition, voluntary. One by one, the meeting of human needs and human problems was mandated by legislation—elementary education, vaccination against certain diseases, sanitary food-processing, protection of women and children from labor exploitation, collective bargaining, certain forms of medical care. In mental health we began with legislation to restrain and incarcerate the madman and have moved on to quite remarkable and even revolutionary legislative requirements. In many states in the United States special education for emotionally disturbed children is required by law, and the regulations for the operation of federally supported community mental health centers spell out quite clearly legal requirements for range of services, equal availability to all residents of the service area, and the maximum and minimum limits of the size of the population to be served.

The first trend line, then, is from private to public, the second from voluntary agreement to legislative requirement. A third

COMMENTARY ON THE COMMENTARY 239

rend is from the special or particular to the general and universal,
both on the part of those who arrange and on the part of those
who are arranged for. As an illustration, we have moved, in
arranging income for the poor, from dealing with a narrowly
bounded, specifically defined category of persons who can be
defined by particular characteristics as the "worthy poor" to
arrangements that are designed for very large groups—in some
cases, theoretically at least, for the total population. Compare
poor relief for the specially defined pauper on the one hand with
unemployment insurance or old-age pensions arranged through
social security mechanisms. And in mental health, where we
began by casting our net (if you will pardon the expression) over
a very small group of persons—those who were willing or forced
to adopt the very highly specialized role of the madman or
maniac—we have continually expanded our area of concern.
Now we deal with the mildly neurotic, the delinquent, the poor
earner, the unhappily married—almost everybody. Indeed, when
we descended on the people of Midtown Manhattan,[1] we could
find only one person in five who did not show some sign of
deviance or distress. The day that used to be predicted by patients in mental hospitals, when there would be more outside than
inside, came a long time ago. So the trend has clearly been from
concern and arrangements for small, highly specialized categories
to large groups, approaching the total population.

The group taking responsibility for making these arrangements
has expanded in a parallel fashion. Initially, management was by
small groups with special responsibilities, such as the vestrymen
of the parish. Then responsibility was generalized somewhat and
vested in larger professional groups. (Mental health became the
responsibility of the medical profession.) Then other professions
began jostling their way in to get a piece of the action. Responsibility was broadened and authority spread even further as general
citizens began to take part in making the arrangements. A refine-

[1] See Leo Srole et al., *Mental Health in the Metropolis: The Midtown
Manhattan Study* (New York: McGraw-Hill, Inc., 1962).

ment is taking place now as we see an insistence on having
consumers represented in the decision-making regarding human
services. In both senses, then—regarding those making the deci
sions and those about whom the decisions are being made—the
trend has been from the special and particular to the general and
inclusive.

The trend from remedial activities to preventive and promotive
activities is also very clear; we have gone from bleeding, cutting
and medicating to inoculating, sanitizing, and educating. Gener
ally speaking, it is the trend from medical care to public health
And it goes even beyond public health. Such indicators as the
World Health Organization definition of health as having physi
cal, emotional, and social components suggests that even the
medical field is moving beyond the medical framework to
broader, more comprehensive social welfare framework. This
trend has been much less clear-cut in the mental health field
although there has certainly been a shift from custodial care of
the chronically disabled to active treatment, early case-finding
and some emphasis on such preventive activity as family life
education.

Finally, we see the trend from local to national—from the town
overseers of the poor to the state or provincial welfare depart
ment to the national welfare program, and from the local alms
house or county workhouse to the state hospital to the commu
nity mental health center, whose program is largely shaped by
federal regulations and supported by federal funds.

These are the trend lines then: private to public, voluntary to
legislated, special to universal, particular to general, remedial to
preventive, local to national. Of course these trends have not been
along a straight line, have not been unambiguous, and, in particu
lar, have not implied mutual exclusiveness. The private coexists
with the public, but the *emphasis* has shifted. Voluntary arrange
ments continue to exist in the midst of those that are planned and
legislated. Local efforts persist; remedial treatment remains ne

only important but necessary. Still, the trend lines are clearly evident, with the center of gravity gradually shifting from the anchor point at one end toward the anchor point at the other.

The trends are, of course, not accidental or random. They reflect what might be termed an environmental or societal "pull." In all industrialized, complex nations, particularly those with strong democratic and egalitarian principles and traditions, the needs of citizens have resulted in a variety of governmental actions to insure some minimum provision of service in a standardized, orderly, manner. Some have referred to this as the development of the "welfare state." However one defines these "pulls," it is quite evident that they are there, most clearly in the form of governmental and, particularly, federal action.

In the beginning I suggested that these five or six trend lines, which are clearly visible, may well reflect an underlying dimension, which may not be so evident. Such a dimension has been specified in the work of Wilensky and Lebeaux. They talk about two different conceptions of social welfare, which they label the *residual* and the *institutional*.

Let me quote their explanation of these two contrasting and often warring conceptions of what social welfare is all about:

> Two conceptions of social welfare seem to be dominant in the United States today: the *residual* and the *institutional*. The first holds that social welfare institutions should come into play only when the normal structures of supply, the family, and the market break down. The second, in contrast, sees the welfare services as normal, "first line" functions of modern industrial society. . . .
>
> The residual formulation is based on the premise that there are two "natural" channels through which an individual's needs are properly met: the family and the market economy. These are the preferred structures of supply. However, sometimes these institutions do not function adequately: family life is disrupted, depressions occur. Or sometimes the indi-

vidual cannot make use of normal channels because of old age or illness. In such cases, according to this idea, a third mechanism of need fulfillment is brought into play—the social welfare structure. This is conceived as a residual agency, attending primarily to emergency functions, and is expected to withdraw when the regular social structure—the family and the economic system—is again working properly. . . .

. . . [The] definition of the "institutional" view implies no stigma, no emergency, no "abnormalcy." Social welfare becomes accepted as a proper, legitimate function of modern industrial society in helping individuals achieve self-fulfillment. The complexity of modern life is recognized. The inability of the individual to provide fully for himself, or to meet all his needs in family and work settings, is considered a "normal" condition; and the helping agencies achieve "regular" institutional status.

While these two views seem antithetical, in practice American social work has combined them, and current trends in social welfare represent a middle course. . . .[2]

It can be seen, then, that the series of trends referred to above bears a considerable resemblance to this formulation. In each case, the movement from one anchor point to another can be thought of as analogous to a movement from what Wilensky and Lebeaux call *residual* to what they call *institutional*. The private, the voluntary, the special, the particular, the remedial, and the local are more or less consistent with a residual formulation; the public, the legislated, the universal, the general, the preventive, and the national anchor points with an institutional formulation.

While there are similarities between Wilensky and Lebeaux's formulations and the trends I've been describing, there are also important differences. First, they limit themselves to the field of

[2] Harold N. Wilensky and Charles N. Lebeaux, *Industrial Society and Social Welfare* (New York: The Free Press, paperback edition, 1965), pp. 138–40.

social welfare and, for the most part, to administrative and policy aspects of this field; and, second, they talk about two different conceptions rather than a continuum. For these reasons, it would seem prudent to introduce a somewhat different terminology for the hypothetical single dimension that underlies the trends I have been discussing. We will therefore name this underlying continuum the *exceptional-universal* dimension.

The *exceptionalist* position is analogous to Wilensky and Lebeaux's residual conception. This outlook perceives social problems and needs for human services as *exceptions* to the general run of affairs—as accidental, unpredictable, arising from special, individual circumstances. At the level of programs or arrangements for service the exceptionalist would hold that such arrangements are outside the range of enduring relationships that are contractual or otherwise part of the public order. Such arrangements are unusual and temporary and, in particular, are *voluntary*, which is to say that they are based on terminable arrangements between individuals and depend on continuously renewed consensus.

The person with a *universalist* outlook, on the other hand, sees social problems as rooted in societal and structural contradictions —as general, regular, and expected; he sees the need to approach the problem with systematic arrangements that are not dependent on individual agreement but are ordered and canonical and have a goal of systemic and structural change that can be institutionalized.

The universalist tends to look more closely at the rule than at the exception; his framework is more often the collective, the group, the social system, whereas that of the exceptionalist is the individual. The exceptionalist is shocked by accidents; the universalist expects the consequences of structural defects. The exceptionalist wants to repair lesions; the universalist wants to prevent injuries. The exceptionalist wants to change attitudes; the universalist acts to change laws. When he goes on an ocean journey, the exceptionalist insists on seaworthy and well-stocked lifeboats, while the universalist requires a precisely accurate compass and radar. In the darkness, the exceptionalist urges each man to light a candle, while the universalist establishes a rule that everyone must contribute to the cost of a generator.

Historical trends in the direction of a universalistic set of arrangements, together with the requirements inherent in both the complexity of the modern metropolis and the emerging patterns of physical, social, and health planning, suggest certain clear guidelines for planning enterprises in the cities of America in 1969 and the immediate years ahead.

To begin with, mental health services must be carried out with a substantial—yes, dominant—role being played by the public agency. They must be carried out within a framework of clearly defined planning structures strongly rooted in relevant and effective legislation. They must be carried out with the explicit aim of providing a coverage program to a total population rather than simply giving isolated services to small, special subgroups suffering from specific disorders. They must be planned and implemented with the involvement and participation of ever-increasing segments of the total population, particularly those from low-income and minority neighborhoods and those who have been or might expect to be consumers of the services. They must be oriented more toward preventive activities rather than being limited to remedial and rehabilitative programs for those who have already fallen victim. They must be organized within the context of a general national consensus about procedures, financing arrangements, and program goals. The boundaries of the mental health system must be carefully delimited but, at the same time, the mental health system must be closely integrated and made interdependent with other human service programs.

I will not extend my remarks in this section any further but will refer the reader back to the essays by Alfred Kahn and David

Vail and recommend a careful re-reading of the thoughtful and sophisticated explications which they have offered.

III. Policy Issues

Three policy issues have been raised that require careful attention: the question of "two-class care"; the problem of manpower and resource distribution; and the issue of medical control.

That there are, in fact, two mental health systems in this country—one of rather good quality for those of us with resources and a second of very poor quality for those of us lacking in resources—has been documented, reviewed, analyzed, and pointed to with alarm by many of us, including a sizable number of the contributors to this book. Going back ten years to Hollingshead and Redlich,[3] we can trace a growing concern and an escalating level of outcry about this situation. Here and there, efforts have been made to correct the situation, but, by and large, the problem has not changed significantly. We still find new mental health centers opening up in general hospitals, whose policies are such that only a token commitment is made to services for the poor, which is not terribly different from the time-worn practice of setting aside "charity beds." While this kind of policy may be tolerable when it is put forth by an institution operating wholly in the private voluntary sphere, it can hardly be considered acceptable when the institution is predominantly financed by tax funds. The question that remains unanswered is this: what *policy* provisions must be established to eliminate two-class care?

Two strategies are beginning to emerge. One, exemplified by the United Auto Workers program, might be called an insurance strategy, which, by equalizing access to fee-paying resources,

---

[3] See August B. Hollingshead and Frederick C. Redlich, *Social Class and Mental Illness* (New York: John Wiley & Sons, Inc., 1958).

hopes to provide equalized access to treatment resources that are judged to be of the highest quality—that is, treatment by a psychiatrist, preferably one in private practice. The second strategy, more amorphous, is based on the idea of broadening the pool of mental health workers and, in the process, building bridges of communication and understanding between the poor community and the mental health facility. Typically, this strategy is put into action by the employment of "indigenous nonprofessional" workers, who provide both liaison and treatment services to the poor community. In a sense, it might be said that the first is an inflationary strategy and the second a strategy of devaluation.

The insurance strategy runs head on into the law of supply and demand in an essentially monopolistic situation. There is a limited supply of psychiatrists, with no elasticity for increasing the supply; an increase in demand brought about by an insurance program only creates a more competitive situation. The field of psychiatric care, which was already a sellers' market, becomes in this way nothing less than a sellers' paradise. The main result one would expect from such an increase in demand is a sharp increase in psychiatrists' fees, for precisely the same reason that a primary result of the introduction of the Medicare program was a rapid increase in physicians' fees.

The indigenous nonprofessional strategy, as it affects the provision of increased services, runs the danger of lowering the quality of service. (The liaison and communicative aspects of this strategy have a different effect, which will be further commented upon.) The "nonprofessional" is typically a person drawn from the poverty community, who is identified as having natural talents for human service work, who is provided with short-term training in basic skills, and who functions in a helping capacity with poor clients. He is often extremely good at his job and in most cases very helpful to clients—more helpful than a psychiatrist could ever be, since the help needed by these clients usually is of a much more practical nature, relating to housing, employment, and welfare problems, than a psychiatrist would be able to give. But, at the same time, there are some clients he tries to help whose *primary* difficulty is chronic, severe emotional disorder— "mental illness," if you will. Typically, the nonprofessional worker will attempt to bring such a client into the professional treatment realm not simply by what used to be known as referral but by active facilitation of his entry through playing the role of expediter. Although the results are considerably better than when the disturbed poor person tries to break into the treatment system on his own, the ministrations of the nonprofessional expediter by no means equalize the access to treatment resources.

One possible by-product of the development of nonprofessional mental health workers, then, is that a "separate-but-equal" care system will develop, which will be in certain infrequent but crucial instances not at all equal, although, of course, it will be better than no community care system for the poor at all.

On the policy level, it would seem that the main task is to neutralize the financial aspects of the very tight supply-and-demand balance. This can be done only by some method of positive discrimination, by building into the regulations governing mental health centers, for example, a provision that they develop intake policies that would tend to *exclude* the middle class and to favor the entry of the poor, while at the same time stressing the maintenance of quality standards. (It was the failure to attend to the latter task, of course, that ruined the state hospital.)

It is only by a heavy public counterbalancing of the private care system that a significant change can be made in the two-track system. In a private enterprise economy it is doubtful that a two-class system can ever be completely abolished (there is reason to doubt that it should be), but it should be possible to bring about a situation somewhat analogous to that of elementary and secondary education, where the public program is dominant and the private program dwindles to a minor arena, available as an alternative choice to those who wish to use it for reasons either of theology or snobbery.

Another way of *naming* the tight supply-and-demand situation is to call it the manpower problem. Again, there is no need to restate the basic dimensions of the problem; they have been outlined in Part Two in several different ways. It would seem to me that there are three questions here that could be solved by appropriate changes in policy, particularly governmental policy.

Professional mental health workers today, particularly psychiatrists and clinical psychologists, are the recipients of enormous quantities of teaching. They are awesomely knowledgeable, armed with an array of skills that would make the average Renaissance man blush with inferiority feelings. Consider the psychiatrist—in a pinch, he could deliver a baby, snip out an appendix, perform a passable urinalysis, diagnose either a dissecting aorta, a tumor in the third ventricle, or an hysterical neurosis, operate an electron microscope, prescribe a bewildering array of drugs, lecture on the complexities of psychoanalytic theory, engage in individual, group, and family therapy, consult with school teachers or policemen, and administer and lead such a complex social system as a ward in a mental hospital. Most clinical psychologists can match the psychiatrist in psychotherapeutic skills and, in addition, can interpret Rorschach tests, run research data through an analysis of variance, teach a course in learning theory or the physiology of hearing and vision, program a computer, manage a manpower training program for the hard-core unemployed, lobby for changes in state medical malpractice legislation, administer social agencies, and "cool out" the underpaid workers in a factory operating in a marginal industry.

Does it make sense to use such fantastically skilled and elaborately trained persons in the role of a clinician, who typically makes use of only a fraction of these skills? The obvious answer is

No. It's clearly not an economical use of manpower. And, in fact, these highly trained professionals are *not* typically used as first-line clinicians. Even those in private practice tend to spend up to half their time in teaching, consulting, and research. And in institutional settings very little of their time is devoted to work with patients. Here we see a classical example of practice racing ahead of theory.

In an effort to fill the *clinical* manpower gap, we spend millions of tax dollars training people who ultimately provide very little clinical service. The problem is that we are *overtraining* a handful of specialists (overtraining, that is, from the point of view of clinical need rather than in any absolute sense) and doing very little training of people who might actually plug the manpower gap that we all keep wringing our hands about.

A parallel issue here is that the tax-supported clinical training programs provide very few persons who provide a substantial amount of direct clinical service in tax-supported settings; they do turn out a fair number, mostly psychiatrists, who go into private practice. In this sense, tax money is being used to subsidize psychiatric care for the well-to-do.

At the opposite end of the scale we provide too *little* training, particularly at intermediate levels. There are sharp jumps in the theoretical level of skills as we move, say, from the psychiatric aide to the psychiatric nurse or to the social worker, or from the social worker to the psychiatrist. In first-class mental health facilities one finds relatively few "subprofessionals"—such as case aides, psychologists with only one or two years of graduate training, etc. There is, then, a *theoretical* ladder of mental health skills with a relatively small number of rungs. Now, in fact, the actual level of skills of various practitioners tends to be unrelated to the theoretical level attributed to them. And the actual number of rungs on the ladder of skills is more than it appears to be. The central issue I am driving toward is that there is no formal or systematic recognition of the gradations in skills and, in particular, there is no provision for intermediate training that would qualify a person to move from one level to another.

In summary, the manpower problem is complicated by three problems related to training: the overtraining of a small number for clinical positions, the tendency of psychiatrists trained with public funds to move into private practice, and the lack of gradations of intermediate training parallel with the many theoretical levels of skills between the completely untrained mental health workers beginning their careers and the most highly trained professionals.

A problem directly related to manpower is that of distribution of resources. Martin Rein accurately and acutely divined the nature of the Boston Mental Health Survey as "distributive research." The utter lack of congruence between the distribution of disturbed persons to different agencies and the distribution of resources to those agencies has been commented on not only by the contributors to this book but by many others who have studied the problem. The tendency for the least-endowed agencies to be flooded and burdened with the greatest numbers of seriously disturbed clients, which was suggested in the Boston data, has also been found in other cities. All of this is, of course, complicated by some of the manpower training problems touched on above.

Michael Amrine's concept of the "mythical doctor" fits right into this issue. It must certainly be obvious to most that, purely because of his very low prevalence in the population, the psychiatrist cannot begin adequately to deal with mental health problems on his own. There are two possible solutions: the psychiatrist can relinquish his special claim to being more equal to the task than others and join as a peer with other disciplines in a broad mental health effort; or he can drastically limit his efforts to unequivocally medical problems, such as organic brain diseases. My guess is that the majority of psychiatrists will ultimately choose the first solution and will move on an equal interdisciplinary footing into nonmedical modes of dealing with what we now call mental illnesses and that a minority will choose to continue being primarily physicians, dealing with the clearly medical component of the mental patient population. The individual psychiatrist will not be able logically to choose both alternatives.

This situation leads to a final policy issue, that of medical control of mental health facilities. This is, in a sense, a subcategory of the more general question of the usefulness and appropriateness of the medical model in the mental health field (which I will deal with in more detail later), but it has additional implications at the policy level. If mental health facilities and particularly the new community mental health centers are, in practice if not in explicit theory, to be viewed as *medical* institutions, which are necessarily under the administrative control of physicians—and with relatively few exceptions this is the general case now—there are certain clear consequences. First, such a policy causes subtractions from the pool of clinical resources by calling for an expensively trained psychiatrist with sharply honed skills to be set to a task for which he is often unprepared either by education, by experience, or by temperament, sometimes with disastrous results. Second, it gives a message to other professionals, particularly psychologists and social workers, that they are in foreign territory and that they can expect to be treated as aliens, honored ones perhaps, but clearly aliens, ineligible for high political office and other privileges of citizenship. I am not arguing in any sense the question of medical responsibility for medical practices and procedures (although I am prepared to argue—and will begin to do so shortly—the issue of the placement of the boundaries that encompass medical practices and procedures). I am raising the question of the reality of the mental health enterprise as an interdisciplinary undertaking. A truly interdisciplinary endeavor cannot logically be placed exclusively under the administrative control of one discipline. There is now a serious danger that a continuation of the policy of medical control of mental health programs and agencies will ultimately lead to a breakdown in the level of interdisciplinary cooperation, which most observers see as an actual or at least a potential strength. Present policies, as they are embedded in a variety of state and federal legislation and regulations, carry the clear assumption that mental health is a medical concern. My own feeling, shared by many others in psychology and social work, is that such policies are no longer tenable and will shortly begin to do more harm than good.

It can be seen that all of these policy questions—arrangements to correct the inferior services given to the poor, reorganization of training to improve the manpower supply, allocation of manpower and financial resources, and medical control—are in some sense variations of the central manpower or personnel issue, in that they raise in various ways the question "Who is to do what to whom?" To which, of course, the answer is "It depends." What "it depends" *on* is what is wrong and what is to be done. Which leads directly to the fourth major question raised by the commentators, the whole problem of conceptualization of mental health problems and mental health services.

IV. Conceptualization Issues

Where does the field of mental health end and other fields of service begin? What is the distinction between the field of mental health and the medical specialty of psychiatry? Is every life situation that is accompanied by anxiety or depression or somatic symptoms of psychogenic origin a mental health problem? Where are we to draw the appropriate lines that will demarcate boundaries? Or are there, in fact, any meaningful boundaries at all?

These are some of the central questions raised particularly by Arnhoff's thoughtful essay on conceptualization problems and

Kahn's wise exposition of the parameters of the planning task, as well as by remarks made by Levinson, Duhl, and Albee. The boundary issue is becoming paramount as we see two contradictory forces at work. First, there is the movement that could be termed "mental health imperialism," the slogan of which might well be "Today schizophrenia, tomorrow the world!" We have seen in past decades manifestations of mental health imperialism in the proliferation of psychiatric diagnoses applied to human problems that in past times have, by consensus, been included within the fields of correction and education. Behavioral manifestations of criminal tendencies are used as criteria for psychiatric categorization, as are straightforward classroom learning difficulties. This movement has recently extended into the treatment as well as the diagnostic aspects of mental health services. Mental health professionals have shown signs of reinventing the settlement house, the Big Brother movement, the group care facility of the child welfare field, and, in some measure, the family service agency.

The opposing force is the resurgence of "medicinism," the return of the white coat, epitomized in the idea of bringing psychiatry back into the mainstream of medical care and the increased emphasis on the general hospital as the logical core of a community mental health program. Here we see an increment in the biological and metabolic elements in care and treatment and the development of virtuosity in the pharmacology of mental health. This represents an isolationist as opposed to an imperialist trend (in terms of diagnostic and treatment modalities, at least, though not usually in terms of the population "belonging to" the mental health professional).

At the etiological level the conceptual issue is whether to choose between viewing situations relevant to mental health as life problems and viewing them as diseases or to distinguish between these two concepts but admit both. At the service level the conceptual issue is more tender and controversial, requiring a choice between assigning services for the emotionally disturbed to the field of medicine and assigning them to the broader field of social welfare. Obviously, any distinction to be made between the field of psychiatry and the field of mental health must hinge on these questions. Psychiatry, as a medical specialty, *must* view its practice as medical practice and its patients as diseased persons.

The problem is that psychiatry as a profession has been reluctant to face up to this dilemma. Most psychiatrists do not wish to follow through on the logic of the implications inherent in such a formulation. Albee, in his insistently rational way, has pointed out that there is much to be done by psychiatrists as *physicians*, and this is obviously true. Consider the number of persons psychiatrically disabled by clear-cut brain dysfunction, by severe psychosomatic disorder, by metabolic deviance, by perinatal trauma, and similar causes. There is an enormous amount of remedial and preventive work to be done that is unquestionably within the boundaries of medical practice.

But the average psychiatrist is not drawn to this type of case. He prefers to deal with patients who are not readily included within the clear-cut boundaries of medical problems, persons whose problems are just as easily cast in social, psychological, semantic, or learning terms and whose treatment requires no particular medical skills. His preferences are shared by a large number of nonpsychiatric professionals—psychologists, social workers, and nurses, particularly. The vaguely bounded area of practice which includes such patients is more and more being labeled "mental health" rather than "psychiatry." Practicing in this field, the psychiatrist is often tempted to define himself as a behavioral scientist or a social scientist. As such, he leaves himself open to the facetious charge of practicing psychology without a Ph.D. from his nonmedical colleagues and to the charge of abandoning his membership in the brotherhood of Aesculapius from his medical friends.

The crucial *fact* we are faced with is that there are millions of troubled persons who cannot be fitted into strictly medical categories but who are nevertheless as likely as not to be considered mental health problems. The category into which they are to be fitted has not as yet been defined, its boundaries have not been set, and their proper place in the total system of human services has not been defined. The crucial conceptual problem to be dealt with is this: what is the problem to which mental health services, particularly the psychotherapeutic services, provide a solution? At this moment in time, the answers are being formulated in more negative than positive terms around the idea of the *medical model* (speaking of treatment) and the *disease model* (speaking of causation). Since that is where we are today, let us consider the problem of the disease model.

THE NEED
FOR A NEW
MODEL

There can be little question that the introduction of the disease model as an explanation for emotionally disturbed behavior represented a tremendous advance in humane treatment and in rational thinking about this problem. The kinds of explanations for which this substituted—such as "possession" or innate defect of one sort or another—gave rise to very little that was beneficial to the disturbed person or that provided any kind of advance in scientific analysis of this category of behavior. As Maurice Chevalier has often said, when asked how he felt about reaching the age of eighty, "Considering the alternative, I am delighted." So, when we begin to feel dissatisfied and fretful about the deficiencies of the disease model in emotional disorder, it is perhaps useful and wise to consider the alternatives, for which it was a useful and beneficial substitute for a century or more.

In my own view, the conceptual difficulties arising from the disease model are most harmful in their secondary rather than their primary effects. The use of analogies related to diseases and to medical procedures involves a set of more or less unquestioned assumptions that interfere with rational thinking about problems, problem-solving procedures, and problem-solving personnel. For example, the assumption that emotional disorder is reflective of a disease process leads to the use of a set of words—"symptoms," "diagnosis," "treatment," "therapy," "patient," "therapist," "prognosis," "nursing," "hospital," and many others—that are prescriptive of certain detailed ways of acting and of not acting. It leads us, for example, to endless quibbling and squabbling about how we should count "cases" for epidemiological studies, what we should use as criteria for the "onset" of the "disease," what "diagnostic" criteria we should use, etc. There is, of course, no answer to these endless questions because the medical terminology we use is, in fact, only metaphorical in nature. If there is in fact *no* disease process in the scientific way that term is ordinarily used, there can be no criteria for determining the onset, no way of establishing reliable diagnostic criteria. One cannot apply epidemiological methods to mental health problems except through a process of metaphorical adaptation.

Another example of the maladaptive use of medical analogies is to be found in the architecture of mental hospitals and mental health centers, where features appropriate to a general medical and surgical institution are transferred and applied thoughtlessly —and very expensively—not because of any particular need but because the medical analogy bears down on the imagination of the architect and the builders and the planners of the building. Oxygen outlets in every room of a mental health center are an outright absurdity. In staffing these institutions, guided by our insistence on thinking in medical terms, we are compelled to hire dozens and dozens of nurses, who are, in a very real sense, superfluous. This is not to attack the usefulness and training of the good modern psychiatric nurse, who is often as skilled and able as the best psychiatrist in the "hospital." Rather, the difficulty arises from the fact that such institutions are usually heavily staffed *not* with trained psychiatric nurses but with medically oriented nurses, who are, in fact, beginners and neophytes in this kind of institution. But, since we call the center a medical institution, it follows that we must staff it with medical nurses.

When we worry about problems of chronicity, we immediately fall into the medical semantic trap and wonder about ways of improving early "case-finding" and referral, precisely as though we were dealing with a definable disease like glaucoma or diabetes. The many studies of the failure of case-finding and referral in mental health problems—one of which was presented in Part One of this book—testify to the uselessness of this kind of formulation.

The disease model, then, is no longer pragmatically useful. It impedes the rational development of services for people in trouble. It adds nothing to our general capacity to understand and to cope with the problems presented by these people. It raises a confusing series of barriers to effective programming—beginning with the fundamental question of medical responsibility and continuing through such issues as architecture, epidemiological research, staffing patterns, "treatment" traditions, and allocation of research and training funds. The manpower crisis in mental health is, in large measure, attributable to our insistence on clinging to the disease model. The logic is that, if emotional disorder is a disease, we must have thousands of doctors and nurses and highly trained "paramedical" personnel to cope with it. Consider how the manpower crisis would be simplified and made quite soluble if the President were to issue an executive order declaring that, for all purposes relating to federal programs, mental illness was no longer to be considered an illness.

The barrier to such an approach, the problem behind the problem, is that we have no satisfactory, thoroughly worked out, widely acceptable alternative to the disease model. Such an alternative, however, is clearly on the verge of being born. Enough people have now begun to think about problems involving emotional disorder in psychological, social, and learning terms to enable us to feel quite safe in predicting that an alternative model is gestating. Meanwhile it is an unfortunate but probably a true fact that the term "mental health problem" is really not at all useful in most instances. No definition of it is available that is widely acceptable. This was true when we were conducting the Boston survey some years ago (several commentators astutely pointed out our deficiencies on this score and the kinds of ambiguity and vagueness that necessarily resulted from those deficiencies) and it is true today. It is only when we skip beyond any generic definition of mental illness as a general phenomenon and concentrate on individual diagnostic categories that we can even keep people from jumping up out of their seats and waving their fists. Unfortunately, even at this level, on the question of psychiatric diagnosis, it is almost impossible to get the kind of agreement between different diagnosticians that would make even specific diagnostic categories useful for scientific discourse and rational program planning.

There is a small core of definable problem entities on which agreement can be reached. These include, certainly, behavior disorders that are directly referable to brain trauma or disease, as well as some of the more severe psychosomatic disorders. They would also include a quantitatively minor set of metabolic and toxic disorders that produce deviant behavior. This set of disorders could be called "mental disease" and few if any would object. One might even find a substantial minority if not an actual majority of mental health professionals (on Mondays, Wednesdays, and Fridays I am counted in their number) who would be willing to count as diseases in the strict sense certain kinds of very severe major mental disorders, characterized, for example, by definable hallucinations and sensory confusion, by extreme deficiencies in cognitive processes, by continually uncontrolled assaultive behavior, by hyperactivity leading to exhaustion, by stuporous states, and by similar "symptoms" indicative of severe and advanced stages of the "diseases" we call schizophrenia and manic-depressive psychosis.

These diseases—I will omit the quotation marks at this point—are usually very disabling, prolonged, and refractory to treatment. Persons so diseased make up the majority of long-term residents of mental hospitals. Such persons are most difficult to endure in family, work, or social settings; they are most costly to the community with respect to their failure to become productive members of society. They make up, in a very real sense, the "hard core" of the mental health problem.

But we must also recognize that such persons, those who might legitimately be defined as being *ill*, as being in need of medical care, as suffering from a disease, make up only a small minority of the many millions of persons who are ordinarily caught up in the broad net of mental health problems as they are usually defined —in very general, inclusive terms. They ordinarily appear in very small numbers in the offices of psychiatrists in private practice; they are relatively scarce in low-fee psychiatric clinics. When they appear in these settings, they are often not able to thread their way through the fine holes in the intake screen. The only kind of mental health facility in which they appear in substantial numbers is the public mental hospital.

The larger group of less severely disordered persons constitutes the daily catch in the mental health waters. And these persons fall outside the realm of any rigorously defined categories of mental diseases. The logical error we make is in dealing with such *non-diseased* persons in the same settings and with the same conceptual terminology that we have constructed for the truly *diseased* person. It is true that they are far more pleasant to deal with, that they tend to get better with gratifying regularity, that they are much more like normal people in their activities of daily living. But these facts are no excuse for evading the logical correction of the logical error that has been made. The solution is first to declare the great majority of persons with mental health problems but no mental disease as being out-of-bounds for the medical field and second to direct at least a substantial proportion of the reluctant psychiatrists and some of their allies back to the problems they are best equipped to deal with: the persons with mental diseases, who are now ordinarily so shamefully neglected.

And the others? They can be managed about as readily in a number of different kinds of social agencies as they can be in medical institutions. One would expect that, once they have been declared no longer the exclusive property of the medicine men, the conceptual ferment now going on will produce not only an appropriate categorization but also an appropriate service program and an appropriate set of service facilities. The mental hospital, after all, was invented scarcely more than a century ago. The new service facility for what we can now only call, rather awkwardly, the nonmedical mental health problem, will be invented in a similar fashion to fit the newly defined need. I am sometimes hopeful that the community mental health center is the Model-T of that institution of the future.

FRETTING ABOUT THE POOR

❦

I. Blaming the Victim

Certainly one of the major tasks in developing an alternative for the disease model will be to explain the excess rate of distress and disorder among the poor. Such an explanation should carry within it implications for service programs that differ substantially from most of the treatment programs we know of today.

In observing the growing interest in the relationship between poverty and mental health, which has been particularly evident over the past seven or eight years, my own mood has ranged from exhilarated gratification through puzzlement to a growing sense of concern and dismay. I see signs that the mental health approach to the problems of the poor is being gradually fitted into the same mold that contains and cripples most other approaches to the poor. The central event in this constraining and crippling process is conceptual or, rather, ideological, what I have called elsewhere *"blaming the victim."* [1] Briefly, "blaming the victim" is an intellectual process whereby a social problem is analyzed in such a way that the causation is found to be in the qualities and

[1] See William Ryan, *Blaming the Victim* (New York: Pantheon Books, in press).

262

characteristics of the victim rather than in any deficiencies or structural defects in his environment. In addition, it is usually found that these characteristics are not inherent or genetic but are, rather, socially determined. They are stigmas of social origin and are therefore no fault of the victim himself. He is to be pitied, not censured, but nevertheless his problems are to be defined as rooted basically in his own characteristics. Some of the common stigmas of social origin that are used to blame the victim are the concept of cultural deprivation as an explanation for the failures of ghetto schools to educate poor and black children and the concept of the crumbling Negro family as a basic explanation of the persistence of inequality between blacks and whites in America today. "Blaming the victim" is differentiated from old-fashioned conservative ideological formulations, such as Social Darwinism, racial inferiority, and quasi-Calvinist notions of the prospering elect. It is a *liberal* ideology.

How is "blaming the victim" rearing its ugly head in the issue of the mental health of the poor? Principally through the introduction of rather narrow, status-oriented notions of social class. Most studies relating emotional disorder to poverty are cast in the framework not of poverty and affluence but of social class. Further, the definitions of social class derive from the work and concepts of W. Lloyd Warner, whose views on social stratification are based primarily on differences in prestige and in lifestyle.[2] In determining the social ranking of the members of a community, his dependent variable is the esteem in which persons are held; and, although the indices that are correlated with that esteem very definitely include income and possession of property, they are more heavily loaded with such questions as educational level, area of residence, kind of home lived in, clubs in which

[2] See W. Lloyd Warner and Paul S. Lunt, *The Social Life of a Modern Community* (New Haven: Yale University Press, 1941); and W. Lloyd Warner, Marchia Meeker, and Kenneth Eels, *Social Classes in America* (Chicago: Science Research Associates, 1949).

membership is held, social cliques belonged to, churches attended, etc. Warner and his students, then, have focused almost exclusively on life-style issues and such concomitant issues as child-rearing practices and values in their definitions of the social strata along which Americans are ordered. The Warner view on social stratification was the dominant one in American sociology for many decades and his view of social class has dominated most thinking about the relationship between poverty and mental health.

II. Money and Power

There are other views about social stratification that have been far less influential but that might in the long run prove more fruitful for understanding the complexities of relationship between class and distress. Max Weber's conception of stratification, for example, which is followed rather closely by C. Wright Mills and others, maintains that there is not one but three dimensions of social ordering.[3] These are *class*—the extent to which one controls property and financial resources and maintains a favorable position in the marketplace; *status*—the manner in which one consumes resources and the extent to which one is accorded social honor (this is the predominant element in Warner's view of social class); and *power*—the extent to which one (or, more commonly, a group of persons, a "party") is able to control and influence the community's decisions.

Now, if one limits one's thinking about relationships between social stratification and emotional disorder to *status* questions (largely disregarding *class* and *power* issues)—and this has certainly been the dominant tendency in the Warnerian type of thinking about this relationship—one starts seeking explanations

[3] See Max Weber, "Class, Status, and Party," in *Social Perspectives on Behavior*, edited by Herman Stein and Richard Cloward (New York: The Free Press, 1958).

in terms of status elements, such as child-rearing practices, values, life style, etc. One is inclined to conclude that the poor are more subject to emotional disorder than the affluent because their patterns of parenting are deficient, their values are different, their time orientation is different and they cannot defer need-gratification, their life styles emphasize violence and sexual promiscuity, they have ego deficiencies as a result of their childhood experiences in the culture of poverty, etc., etc. One hears and sees these kinds of formulations more and more frequently in mental health settings. I fear that an ideology is developing in which the mental health problems of the poor (which one might reasonably have expected would be related to poverty) are being analyzed through status-oriented formulations of class differences, with the result that these problems are being conceptually transformed into one more category of intrapsychic disorder. The consequences of such transformations are predictable. The evidence that appears to relate disorder to environmental circumstances is being rapidly assimilated to preexisting patterns of intrapsychic theorizing and the status quo is being maintained—which, after all, is the purpose of ideology.

I will be the first to admit that this kind of ideological assimilation is very easy to do. On re-reading Part One of this book, the original report of the Boston survey, I was able to detect quite a few times when I came very close to making this kind of formulation in a very blatant manner. I must confess that I was tempted to edit out some of these phrases—patronizing references to the "disadvantaged"—and unspoken assumptions about cultural differences.

When one focuses on status and life style as explanatory variables, one omits at the same time the other elements that determine social stratification—power and money. Lack of money as a cause of emotional disorder can be conceptualized through the mediating concept of stress. Stresses relating to lack of money—poor and crowded housing, nutritional deficiencies, medical neglect, unemployment, and similar events—have been found as correlates of disorder rather regularly. Moreover, there is evidence that certain kinds of stressful events, such as illness, which can be merely inconvenient for the well-to-do, are often disastrous for the poor. Some of Dohrenwend's recent work contains some intriguing ideas on the possible relationship between poverty, stress, and emotional distress and disorder.[4] He sets forth the hypothesis that reaction to stress is ordinarily cyclical and time-limited and that most emotional symptomatology evidenced in such reaction is temporary. A prevalence study at a given point in time, then, would tend to include substantial numbers of such temporary stress reactions. If one assumes that stresses in the lives of the poor are both more prevalent and more severe than those in the lives of the more prosperous, one would expect that, at a given point in time, the poor as a group would exhibit more stress reactions and would therefore demonstrate a higher prevalence of emotional disorder. This is one example of the way in which the class-oriented method of dealing with stratification, which is to say the money-oriented way, can be introduced into the process of theorizing about the relationship between poverty and mental health.

The third leg of the stratification stool—power—can be dealt with principally through the mediating concept of self-esteem. There is an overwhelming array of theoretical and empirical literature suggesting that self-esteem is a vital element in mental health and, further, that self-esteem is based on a sense of competence, an ability to influence one's environment, a sense of mastery and control over events and circumstances that affect one's life. These are psychological terms that are readily translatable into the sociological concept of power as used by Weber. To the extent that a person is powerful, then, he is more likely to be

[4] See Bruce P. Dohrenwend, "Social Status, Stress, and Psychological Symptoms, *American Journal of Public Health* 57, no. 4 (April 1967): 625–32.

what we call mentally healthy; to the extent that he is powerless, he is likely to be lacking in this characteristic.

The functional relationship between the exercise of power, feelings of self-esteem, and mental health has been empirically observed in a number of settings—civil rights demonstrations, block organization projects, and even, according to some, in ghetto disorders.

There are, then, relationships to be found between mental health phenomena and issues of money and power that are direct —more direct than the secondary kinds of relationships hypothesized between mental health and social status and life style. The major difference, however, is in program implications. If one makes the assumption that the relevant variable is status, one tends to work on changing the characteristics of the individual—his life style, his values, his child-rearing practices, or the effects of the child-rearing practices of his parents. If on the other hand one makes the assumption that the relevant variables are class—i.e., money—and power, one tends to work toward changing the environment, toward developing programs of social change rather than individual change.

I am dismayed and concerned that we in the mental health field are moving more and more toward a narrow view of status issues, which will permit us to conduct business as usual—focusing on changing the person—and avoid the broader view of class and power issues that would oblige us to alter our methods and start putting our resources into the business of social change.

SUGGESTIONS
FOR A NEW
AGENDA
※

What should be the new agenda for mental health? No individual can decide. Nor can any dozen individuals, even the dozen so prolific with agenda items who wrote this book. We must set to the task in large numbers, individually and in groups. As long as I'm up, permit me to list—as a way of summarizing the previous pages—some of the issues that are my candidates for top priority consideration in the formulation of a program.

1. What is to become of the mental health center? Can it develop sufficient flexibility and a close enough relationship with its community to both keep its promises and fulfill its promise?

2. When and how are we going to begin investing in research and programs that are preventive in nature?

3. What policies and strategies can be employed to ensure mental health planning in complex urban areas—planning of a sufficiently universalistic nature to be effective?

4. What strategies can be developed, beyond the insurance and indigenous nonprofessional approaches, that will ensure equal shares in mental health services for the poor?

5. How can our training programs be reorganized and, even more important, be drastically more differentiated, so that we can

268

begin to meet manpower demands realistically by a multiple-skill-level approach?

6. How can we accelerate the conceptualization processes that will provide us with useful alternatives to the disease model and the medical model?

7. How can we stimulate new programs of research and demonstration that will confront the mental health problems of the poor in realistic terms—that is, in terms of money, power, and social change?

8. How can we ensure a rational distribution of resources among the total array of human service agencies?

These are some of the directions in which I would like to see our thinking move.

REFERENCES

Dohrenwend, Bruce P. "Social Status, Stress, and Psychological Symptoms," *American Journal of Public Health* 57, no. 4 (1967): 625–32.

Hollingshead, August B., and Redlich, Frederick C. *Social Class and Mental Illness.* New York: John Wiley & Sons, Inc., 1958.

Ryan, William. *Blaming the Victim.* New York: Pantheon Books, in press.

Srole, Leo; Langner, Thomas; Michael, Stanley; Opler, Marvin; and Rennie, Thomas. *Mental Health in the Metropolis: The Midtown Manhattan Study.* New York: McGraw-Hill, Inc., 1962.

Warner, W. Lloyd, and Lunt, Paul S. *The Social Life of a Modern Community.* New Haven: Yale University Press, 1941.

Warner, W. Lloyd; Meeker, Marchia; and Eels, Kenneth. *Social Classes in America.* Chicago: Science Research Associates, 1949.

Weber, Max. "Class, Status, and Party." In *Social Perspectives on Behavior*, edited by Herman Stein and Richard Cloward. New York: The Free Press, 1958. (Reprinted from Max Weber, *Essays in Sociology*. Translated by H. H. Gerth and C. Wright Mills. New York: Oxford University Press, 1946.)

Wilensky, Harold N., and Lebeaux, Charles N. *Social Class and Mental Illness*. New York: John Wiley & Sons, Inc., 1958.